A GUIDE TO SURGICAL ASSISTING

DR LEETON C. HOCKING

Published in Australia by Dr Leeton C. Hocking

First published in Australia 2025
This edition published 2025

Cover design, typesetting: WorkingType (www.workingtype.com.au)

ISBN: 978-1-7644282-1-7 (pbk)
978-1-7645125-4-1 (ebook)

Cover image: Drs Leeton Hocking and Russell Dalton
with scrub nurse Ann Resgonia

FOREWORD

As a medical student, my earliest lessons were in anatomy. Later, I observed the complexity of decision-making at the bedside. But what struck me most in the operating theatre was seeing a surgeon and assistant work together – seamless, instinctive, almost like a dance built on rhythm, trust, and respect.

As a surgical fellow, I had the privilege of learning from Dr Leeton Hocking. His generosity and insights remain some of the most important lessons of my career. He showed me that surgery is not only about technical skill but about humility, respect, and the value of partnership. To now see him share this wisdom in these pages is a privilege.

This book speaks to all who step into theatre. For the student, it offers permission to be present and to learn. For the doctor in training, it provides a guide to refining this partnership. For the surgical assistant, it is a recipe book of practical instruction. And for the surgeon, it gives insight into how an effective assistant can lift the performance of you both.

There are many texts on anatomy and instruments, but few on the art of surgical assisting. Here, Dr Hocking distils a lifetime of experience – absolute gold for the budding student, the training doctor, the professional assistant, and the surgeon alike.

Dr Madeleine Ward

Gynaecological Surgeon

CONTENTS

INTRODUCTION & ACKNOWLEDGEMENTS

After over 43 years of medical practise, I have been asked by several of my colleagues to share my experience and produce a guide to surgical assisting. This request has especially come from young doctors who are either in training or others at various stages of their careers and are taking on surgical assisting.

After several years as an HMO in the hospital system I have been a general practitioner with a special interest in surgery. I have only practised in Australia but much of what I have included here will possibly apply elsewhere as well. My time has been spent equally in consultative general practice and hospital surgical assisting but recently has been confined entirely to surgical assisting. Over the years, I have assisted dozens of specialist surgeons and hope, in some helpful way, to pass on some of the experience that I have had.

You might ask why a guide to surgical assisting is really needed. There are post graduate nursing degrees provided by some universities for this, but as far as I can ascertain there aren't any practical guideline books written by anyone who has spent so much of their career in surgical assisting. Surgical students, residents and registrars get trained in surgical technique, so what's so special about surgical assisting? Surgical assisting is a unique skill. Specialist surgeons and senior registrars are often not very good assistants as their roles are entirely different to that of an assistant. Of course, as a surgical assistant, it is possible to get by just standing there and doing what you're told, but this doesn't really help the specialist surgeon and certainly won't give any satisfaction or pride to the assistant. Surgical assistants who have pride in their role and do that bit more are generally in high demand.

This guide should prove useful to medical students, HMO's, registrars, nurses, doctors who may occasionally be called on to assist in theatre and those that may intend to make surgical assisting a large part of their career. ***It is not a textbook of surgical technique as there are plenty of these already available,*** and much of this is learnt first-hand on the job. A few basic surgical skills are required to start with, and these will be discussed later. Some areas will be familiar, and some will be informative. I hope the reader will choose that which is most helpful, especially when starting off in this fulfilling and, maybe initially somewhat daunting, career of surgical assisting.

Nothing really teaches better than experience, but hopefully I can pass my experience on to assist those starting their careers in this rewarding and satisfying area of medical practice.

ACKNOWLEDGEMENTS

I would like to express my appreciation to the following:

- Dr Maddy Ward, who suggested that I write this book in the first place and for her ongoing motivation, suggestions and assistance, particularly in reading the draft and offering appropriate ideas and for providing the foreword.

- The staff of the operating theatres of St John of God Hospital Ballarat, Ballarat Day Procedure Centre & Epworth Hospital Geelong for allowing and assisting me in photographing the instruments and equipment.

- Dr Michael Bardsley for the diagrams of the modified Western knot. (All other sketches are my own attempts based on my technique).

- Mr Phil Price from Ecolab for provision of and permission to use their surgical Rub Poster

- My wife, Jo (Practice Manager & Manager of our billing practice "Surgical Assist") for the segment regarding billing, and for allowing me the time and putting up with my cursing and annoyance at the computer and my drawing attempts.

- All my colleagues over the years, many who have already retired. Some have already passed away. The surgeons, anaesthetists, nursing and other theatre and hospital staff, general practitioners and their staff and all the other specialists. The students who have asked pertinent questions and forced me to challenge and justify my knowledge and beliefs. They have all taught me so much.

- My patients, many of whom I've cared for and experienced their ups and downs over my entire career. They too have taught me so much.

PHILOSOPHY & WHY BECOME A SURGICAL ASSISTANT?

Some of us don't have a lot of choice and may be called upon to assist infrequently. Others may be required to do this as part of their training. Meanwhile many of us who love the challenges of consultative type medicine but also love the "hands on" approach of surgery, choose to combine this with the regular part of our career. Some choose to do surgical assisting as their full-time career.

Surgical assisting can be an extremely rewarding career (both in pride and satisfaction as well as financially).

To get down to the "nitty gritty" .... The role of the surgical assistant is really to **make the role of the specialist surgeon as smooth and easy as possible.** (some cynics would say "to make the surgeon look good"). To do this, the surgical assistant must really be a "jack of all trades" and be aware of most, if not all of the dynamics involved. This includes relationships with theatre staff, ward staff, reception staff, knowledge of equipment, being continually vigilant regarding the whole environment as well as having basic (at least) surgical and procedural skills.

BASIC SURGICAL SKILLS REQUIRED

There are a few basic surgical techniques that are needed. When I was a medical student way back last century, these were learnt before we even graduated. Nowadays this is not always taught at undergraduate levels at medical school and must be "acquired" on the job so to speak.

Also, surgical approaches to operations have changed markedly from being predominantly open procedures, through endoscopic approaches (laparoscopies were just starting when I was a student and I remember the professor of surgery telling us that it would never take off and that you'd end up killing too many patients with this approach), and now with robotic assisted surgery with its own unique skill requirements. It is not uncommon for experienced assistants to "close up" after the main procedure is completed. Detailed knowledge is not necessary and much is fortunately learnt with ongoing experience.

Minimal surgical skills needed to start with are:

- Instilling local anaesthetics (and some regional blocks).
  In addition to the anaesthetic provided by the anaesthetist, it is not uncommon to supplement this with local anaesthesia or regional blocks. It is not uncommon for the surgeon or assistant to administer these, so a safe knowledge of dosages and techniques is needed.
  (see appendix for basic local and regional anaesthetic instructions)

- A basic knowledge of common surgical instrument nomenclature.
  (see appendix for descriptions of commonly used basic surgical instruments)

- Suturing - Interrupted, continuous, subcuticular and mattress (vertical and horizontal)
  (see appendix for basic choice of suture, needle and suturing instructions)

- Knot tying – both instrument and hand including one hand and Aberdeen type knot.
  (see appendix for basic knot tying)

- Bladder catheterisation
  (see appendix for bladder catheterisation instructions)

- A sound knowledge of cardiopulmonary resuscitation.
  This is occasionally required, and the surgical assistant will invariably be involved.
  All practising doctors must have a sound knowledge and experience in this. In Australia at least, all practising doctors must undergo regular "refresher" courses as a part of their ongoing re-registration.

More recent developments such as "robotic" assisted surgery are increasing in popularity. Whilst I have been trained in this technique, I realise and emphasise that the basic principles of surgery (and assisting) still apply here. I have not gone into the specific features of robotic assisted surgery in this publication.

BEFORE THE PATIENT ENTERS THE OPERATING THEATRE

The surgical assistant's role really commences here.

You must ensure that you are already accredited to practise at the particular hospital or facility.

Be punctual (arrive early), but don't display annoyance if there are unavoidable delays.

Hopefully you will know the specialist surgeon already and it is also important to introduce yourself to the surgical staff, including the scrub nurse, the scout nurse, the anaesthetist and anaesthetic nurse, the theatre technicians and anyone else involved. Try to remember names (not all that easy, but some theatres have everyone identified on a whiteboard).

Try to have an idea of what surgical procedures are booked beforehand and you may need to refresh up a bit on the anatomy relevant to the procedure. It is important to anticipate what might be involved. Anticipation comes up frequently as a requirement of a good surgical assistant.

When the patient is either in the pre-op area (ward or anaesthetic room) it is important to introduce yourself to them and try to ensure that they understand what is about to happen to them, check for allergies, take a very brief history (to ensure there aren't any important medical issues that might have been missed and as you may have to write up a discharge history), check that the consent document is present, complete and correct (some surgeons turn up at the last minute and the consent may not have been completed) and if appropriate mark the side of the procedure on the patient. Don't spend ages doing all of this and don't get in the way of sometimes what appear to be cranky nurses or anaesthetists. Remember your role is to ensure it all goes as smoothly as possible. Be courteous, but don't be intimidated. Remember also it's about mutual respect.

Pass on any concerns that you may have discovered to the anaesthetist, surgeon or scrub nurse if relevant.

IN THE OPERATING THEATRE BEFORE THE OPERATING STARTS

Try to get an overview of the layout of the operating theatre.

Remember certain areas are sterile - especially the instrument table. Keep a distance from this and don't wander back and forth between the patient and this. The scrub nurse is (justifiably) very protective of this.

Check where the tower for endoscopic and other equipment is and familiarise yourself with the basic functions. (a theatre technician may not always be present or available when adjustments are necessary).

Keep out of the anaesthetist's area as much as possible. The anaesthetist too is (justifiably) very protective of their equipment.

It is often best to wear a surgical mask once the instrument equipment has been opened.

If you have assisted with this procedure before then offer any advice on any special needs such as certain instruments that may be required in this particular case.

When the patient is brought in, offer to assist with transfer onto the operating table. Also assist with correct positioning for the procedure. If you're unsure check with the surgeon re their requirements. The anaesthetist and theatre tech will often know the correct positioning (but not always) and may ask you.

Assist with the final patient check *"Time Out"* in most Australian Hospitals.

BASIC HAND SCRUB TECHNIQUE, GOWNING & GLOVING, MAINTAINING STERILITY

In my day, this was taught as an undergraduate medical student, but this may not be the case nowadays. Also depending on a doctor's experience, this may not have been really taught at all or may have been forgotten. If you are unsure, ask a senior theatre nurse to guide you through this. Don't be too proud to ask. It is best to learn it correctly in the first place and you will continue to do it correctly throughout your career.
(see appendix for basic scrub technique)

Similarly, gowning and gloving may or may not have been taught. I still see young final year medical students as well as some experienced doctors who really have never been taught this. Sometimes the scrub nurse will assist you in this, but this occurs less and less nowadays, and you are expected to do it yourself. Again, don't be too proud to ask for instruction if you are unsure.
(see appendix for basic gowning and gloving technique)

Once you have "gowned and gloved" remember that the sterile area is between your chest and your lower abdomen (and as one of my colleagues repeatedly states, "this space gets narrower with age!"). Resist the temptation to adjust your mask, eye wear, or to cover your mouth when coughing, scratch your nose etc, and keep your hands within the sterile area. If you don't know where to put your hands, then cross your arms across your chest, or lay them on the sterile area of the patient. If you inadvertently breach sterility, then admit it and it can usually be easily corrected.

PREPARING AND DRAPING

This too is a very specific technique, which becomes increasingly obvious with experience.

It is usually the surgeon, the assistant, and/or the scrub nurse that do this.

Firstly, the prep needs to be applied. This is generally done by starting with the immediate surgical area and working outwards towards an appropriate margin. (the exception to this is when the site of the procedure is not deemed as clean, such as rectal or vaginal surgery - in which case this will be prepped last). The extent and type of the prep will depend upon the surgery being performed, the site (don't use alcohol-based preps in the vagina for example - the patient will not thank you - yes, I did it once a long time ago), and whether the patient has any allergies to certain chemicals.

A warning also is to avoid picking anything up or touching anything on the scrub nurse's table unless you have their permission (I was once told that I'd have my "expletive" fingers cut off if I did that again). Also don't hassle the scrub and scout nurse whilst they are doing their "count" of instruments. Be patient and wait until they are ready to commence. Similarly ensure that you check with the anaesthetist and the theatre technician that it's OK to start prepping. (Yes, I've been admonished by an anaesthetist for being too eager and splashing prep on his delicate hands as he was repositioning an IV access).

Draping too is a learned process, and you may do this with the surgeon or be expected to do it with the scrub nurse if the surgeon is not in the room.

Whilst all this may sound a bit intimidating, remember that everyone is a bit tense during these procedures (some more than others), don't take criticism personally, but you don't need to tolerate inappropriate abuse. If this occurs, then sort this out with the offender after the procedure is finished and in an appropriate private environment. Remember that it's about mutual respect. Fortunately, such behaviour has improved markedly over the years.

ONCE THE OPERATING STARTS

Remember that it takes very little effort to be courteous and respectful of all members of the team. "Please" and "thank you" often go a long way. Respect and courtesy are a two-way encounter, and some people sadly lack these basic skills. Others are generally quite good at it but "drop the ball" somewhat under pressure. Egos are often quite strong and evident in the operating theatre environment. Not infrequently the surgical assistant finds themselves in a particularly tense environment and can often assist in diffusing some of the conflict. This is not easy especially when you're just starting, but being aware of this and sometimes appropriate intervention can be most helpful. It's important to get the operation done safely, and appropriately first and then sort out the conflicts. There is no place for fighting (even verbal) during an operation. Patient outcomes are generally better when the whole theatre team feels "psychologically safe" to speak up if they feel that an issue has arisen. Remember too that people working under extreme stress won't perform as well and if they feel that they are being disrespected or abused, they certainly won't defend you if something really goes wrong.

Noise and increasing chatter in the theatre can be most distracting to the surgeon. It is important for the surgical assistant to be aware of this and maybe to ask the nurse in charge to politely ask for less noise. There is a time and place for chatter, and whilst it is quite a pleasant social encounter in theatre, there are times when you need to keep quiet and concentrate and times when appropriate jokes, banter and other talk is quite acceptable.

Appropriate encouragement from the assistant can also be helpful, and even appropriate subtle suggestions often delivered in a question format such as "would this work?" or "I've seen this done" can sometimes help. This clearly depends upon the experience of the specialist surgeon and the assistant, as well as their relationship. Diplomacy is very important. This is all part of building a healthy culture within the surgical team.

Throughout the procedure technically the best assistance that can be provided is **anticipation**. It is important to try to think like the specialist surgeon and anticipate what they are trying to do and assist where possible. This may be technically in the operating or by simply asking the scrub nurse to have another piece of equipment available for use shortly. Again, this type of anticipation develops with increasing experience and confidence.

Technically, the following points are worth noting:

- Maintaining the surgical field of focus: with laparoscopic type procedures - ensure that the camera view is in focus, clear of condensation, upright and centred in the middle of the screen. In these and open procedures try not to cross the field with your hands or instruments.

- Keeping the operating field clear: using suction or dabbing where appropriate.

- Accepting, requesting and passing of surgical instruments: Ask politely, accept, pass and return the instruments to the scrub nurse in a safe fashion - guarded needles, handles first with sharp instruments etc. The latter are best deposited into a dish rather than directly into the recipient's hand. Generally, avoid taking or replacing instruments from and to the scrub nurse's table (unless you have explicit permission) and if returning instruments, replace them to where they belong on the table.

- Maintaining a neat operating area: Try to keep this clear of instruments not in immediate use, (used packs and swabs, used sutures and needles etc.), but avoid doing this at the expense of distracting the specialist surgeon.

- Speaking up: Speak up if you are unsure, if you lose traction on an instrument out of view, if the patient is breathing up or moving, or if you see or anticipate a problem.

- Dealing with complications: Remain calm and in focus, maintain the view and maybe call for further assistance.

- As time goes on, a good surgical assistant will take on increasing responsibility (as the specialist surgeon and nursing staff realise and appreciate their competence and experience).

- When the procedure is completed (the surgeon has often left the operating room), it's a good idea for the assistant to help in applying dressings, removing catheters, drapes etc and assist in getting the patient off the operating table. A simple thank you to the team also goes a long way.

OPERATION NOTES & DISCHARGE SUMMARIES

Not infrequently the surgical assistant may be required to complete these.

Usually, the specialist surgeon will either dictate, type or handwrite operation notes, but sometimes these may not be typed or otherwise available immediately (especially for the recovery room staff). In this case it usually sufficient that the assistant completes some documentation (usually on a hospital provided proforma) with the following details:

Date, Surgeon name, Anaesthetist name, Surgical Assistant name, procedure(s) performed, with brief description of findings, procedure, (for the latter I usually write *"as above and see typed notes for details"* or *"typed notes to follow"*), estimate blood loss and post operative orders. The latter follows along the lines of what reportable observation should be communicated to the surgeon and any special orders such as DVT prevention, dressings, sutures, tubes, drains, catheters etc. Pathology request slips may need to be completed by the assistant. Also, the appropriate item numbers for billing should be documented (always check with the specialist surgeon).

Post operative analgesia is generally (but not always) written up by the anaesthetist but may be left to the surgeon or surgical assistant. Other medications such as those for DVT prevention, patient's regular medications, or special requirements such as antibiotics are frequently the responsibility of the surgical assistant. Check with the specialist surgeon.

Post operative care is otherwise the responsibility of the specialist surgeon.

If the specialist surgeon requires you to complete discharge documentation, then again this will usually be on a hospital proforma. It is important to keep this succinct and relevant. This should include reason for admission, relevant other medical problems, allergies, brief history of presenting complaint, procedures, post operative course, and follow up arrangements.

GETTING PAID

After all this hard work and preparation, you clearly need to be remunerated appropriately.

In Australia, you will need a provider number for Medicare payments, a PRODA (Provider Digital Access) account, an ABN (Australian Business Number) and be registered as a provider with the appropriate health funds. Some assistants accept the Medicare and health fund payments as full payment, and some charge an out of pocket or gap fee to the patient. It is important that the patient is aware of these financial costs prior to their procedure and written, informed financial consent is strongly recommended. If you are going to accept the Medicare rebate only this makes the billing quite simple, but you will only receive 75% of the Medicare determined schedule fee. This payment can be quite low. Including billing to the private health funds brings this up to the schedule fee and sometimes higher.

You can choose to do this billing yourself (this can be quite time consuming and complicated) or you can employ the services of special billing companies who (for a percentage fee) offer this service. What they charge and provide varies considerably and it is important to investigate this thoroughly.

In Australia, the Australian Medical Association recommends that the surgical assistant receives 20% of the specialist surgeon's total fee which may include any gap payment if you chose to add this. Unfortunately, the surgical assistant is always the last to be paid (after the specialist surgeon, the anaesthetist and the hospital). This can take considerable time, especially if the surgeon's billing practice is quite slow, or if Medicare rejects any surgical item number or combination of item numbers being claimed.

If you are charging a gap, it is advisable to recoup this before the procedure, as this can be overlooked by the patients after the procedure. This will also help keep your bad debts to a bare minimum. Therefore, it is important to try to have all the details of the operating list and patient contacts well before the day of the surgery. This requires a good working relationship with the specialist surgeon and their staff.

This can be quite financially rewarding if set up appropriately.

(Refer to appendix for a guide to setting up private billing)

FINAL THOUGHTS AND SUGGESTIONS

As previously mentioned, the above applies to the current situation in Australia, but much of it will be relevant to other areas.

Surgical assisting is a special skill, far removed and advanced from what many think it involves.

It is stimulating, and both professionally and financially rewarding. The operating theatre complex can also be quite a social and enjoyable environment.

It can appear to be intimidating when starting out and challenging at times. Egos and personalities play a big role. Like all areas of medicine, it can be stressful as well. With time and experience it becomes much less daunting.

At the end of the day however it is an essential service to assist the specialist surgeon and the rest of the team in providing an efficient service and hopefully leading to the best possible outcomes for our patients.

APPENDIX

This section provides some basic information and instructions. For many, the information will be well known, and not needed, but for others who may have had limited exposure to surgical procedures, or may have done so a long time ago, some of this information may be of assistance.

BASIC LOCAL ANAESTHESIA INSTRUCTIONS

Comprehensive instruction in this is beyond the scope of this book, but certain basics are required of a surgical assistant. Regional blocks will need to be learnt specifically as needed.

Remember to ***ALWAYS CHECK WITH THE ANAESTHETIST BEFORE INSTILLING THESE*** as, for example, they may have already used some regional block or intravenous effusion which could lead to toxicity if further local anaesthetic is given. They will usually tell you if you can use the local anaesthetic and the dose that you can use.

Maximum safe doses of anaesthetics (these are not necessarily evidence based and are suggestions from textbooks, experience and pharmaceutical companies only):

- Depend on vascularity of the injection site
- Depend on health (including possible allergies) of the patient

- Depend on the weight of the patient
- Depend on the medications (including General anaesthesia)
- Can be cautiously increased in the presence of adrenaline (vasoconstrictor)
- (note – avoid using adrenaline at anatomical sites with end arteries such as digits, penis and pinna due to the risk of ischaemia distal to the injection).

Each local anaesthetic has its own maximum safe dose. The maximum safe volume given therefore depends upon the percentage solution and then the recommended max mg/kg.

A percentage solution is defined as the number of grams of solute per 100ml final volume. Hence a **1% solution = 10mg/ml** (remember this and the calculations are easy).

e.g.

- max safe dose of Lignocaine is 3mg/kg body weight (and from above 1ml of 1% = 10mg)
- max safe dose of Bupivicaine is 2mg/kg body weight
- max safe dose of Ropivacaine is 3mg/kg body weight

The above is a guide only and depends upon the variables mentioned above...always check if in doubt.

REMEMBER TO ALWAYS ASPIRATE BEFORE INJECTING TO ENSURE THAT THE NEEDLE HAS NOT GONE INTO A BLOOD VESSEL.

COMMONLY USED SURGICAL INSTRUMENTS

There is a very large number of surgical instruments in common use. Large volumes have been published about these. Understanding and remembering the naming of these can initially be quite daunting. To further complicate this, many instruments that are the same or very similar have multiple names - sometimes with numerous eponymous names or descriptive names. These names are also often used in an inter-changeable way and are not always used strictly correctly. The way in which they are named and used is often determined by the surgeon you are working with and the institution at which you are working. Some purists will be pedantic about the (often subtle) differences and hence nomenclature. Each instrument has its own application.

This is not in any way a comprehensive discussion of all the instruments in use but is a broad generalisation with samples included to assist in recognising and naming some of the more commonly used instruments that the surgical assistant may encounter and use. Many more instruments may be encountered with further experience and exposure. Photos shown here are all original (with all their patina of age and use) and taken from within the operating theatre.

One way to categorise surgical instruments (grouping similar types) is as follows:

Grasping: Ratcheted

Littlewoods & Morrisons forceps (virtually the same except for tips)

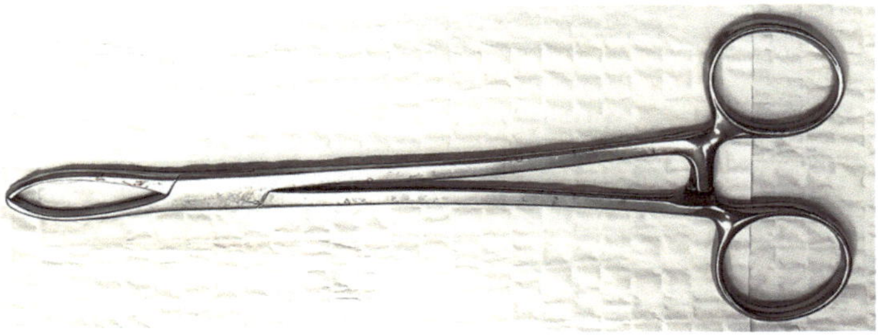

Allis forceps

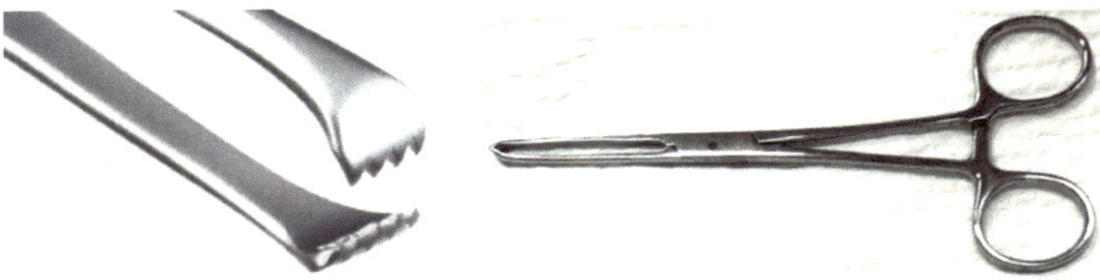

Babcock forceps

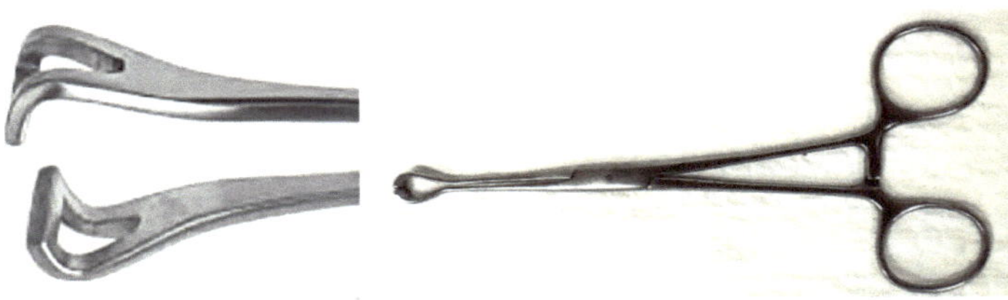

Sponge Holding (Rampley's)

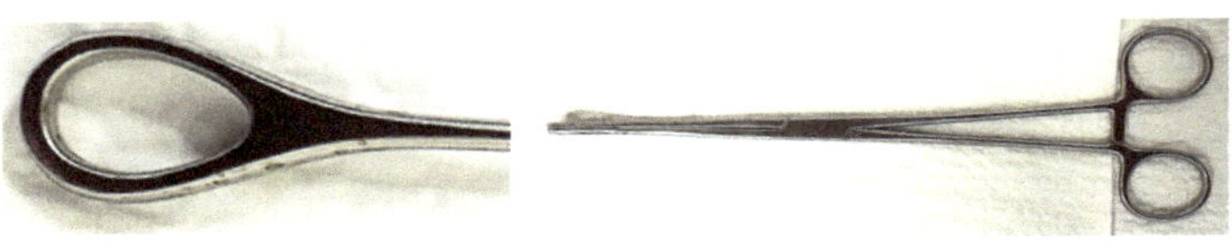

Kochar forceps (straight or curved)

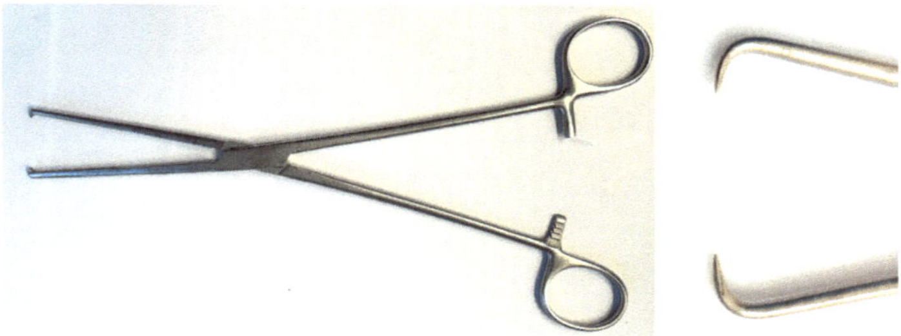

Vulsellum

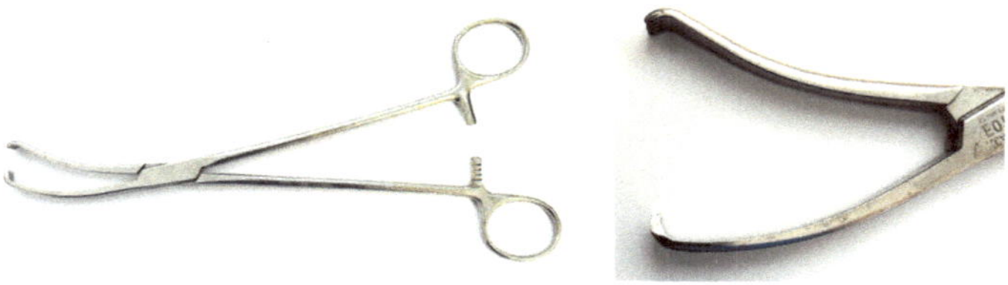

Tenaculum

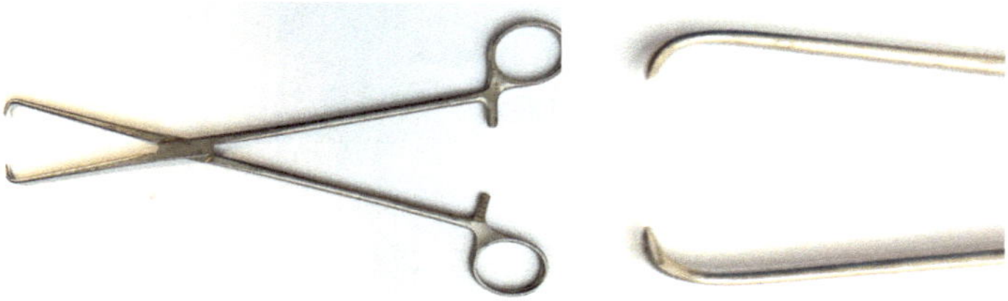

Non-Ratcheted

De Bakey forceps (non-toothed - various sizes)

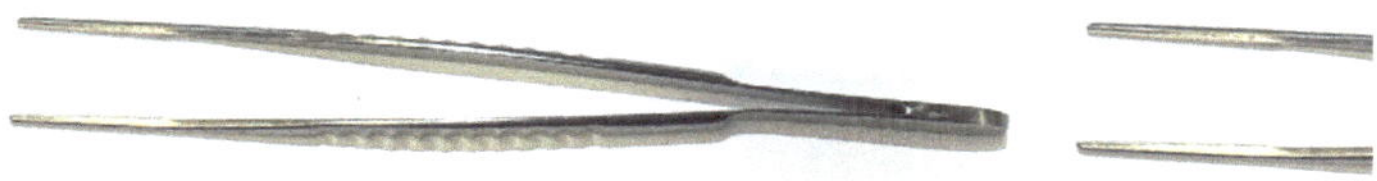

Bonney's forceps (heavy toothed)

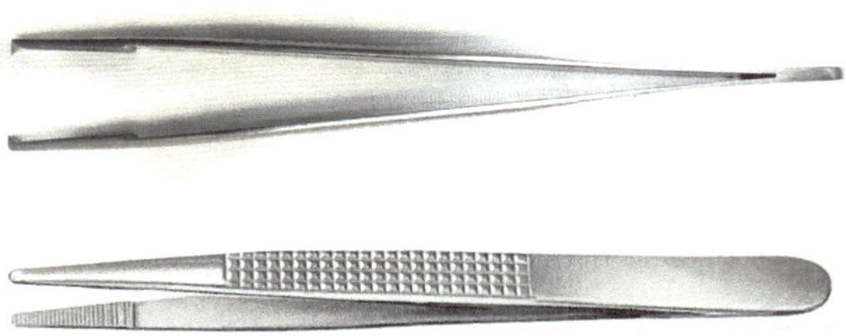

Gillie's forceps (light toothed)

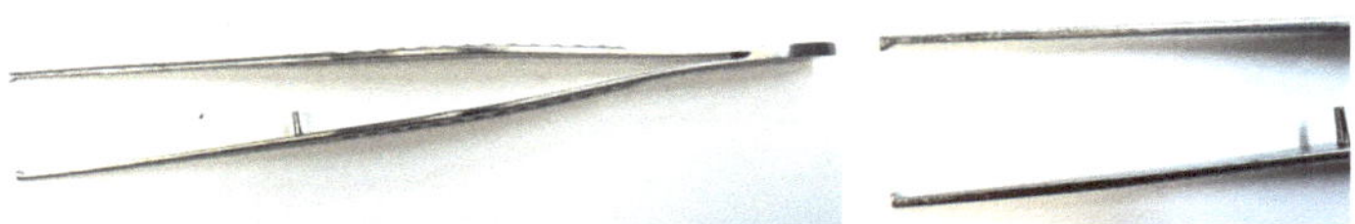

Adson's forceps (light, toothed and non-toothed)

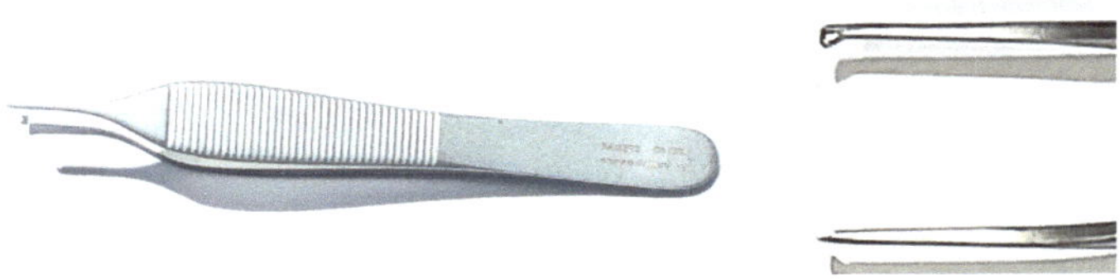

Mayo - Russian Forceps

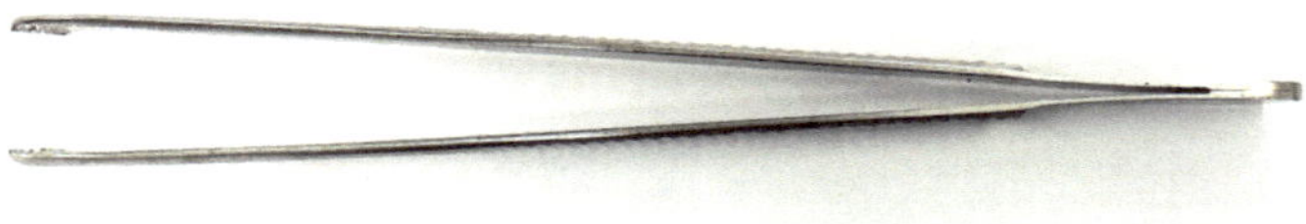

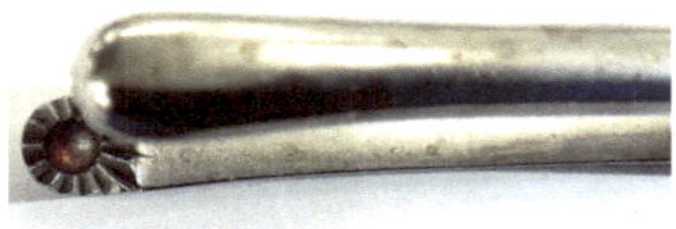

Haemostatic forceps

Spencer Wells, Mosquito etc (curved and straight) differ in size

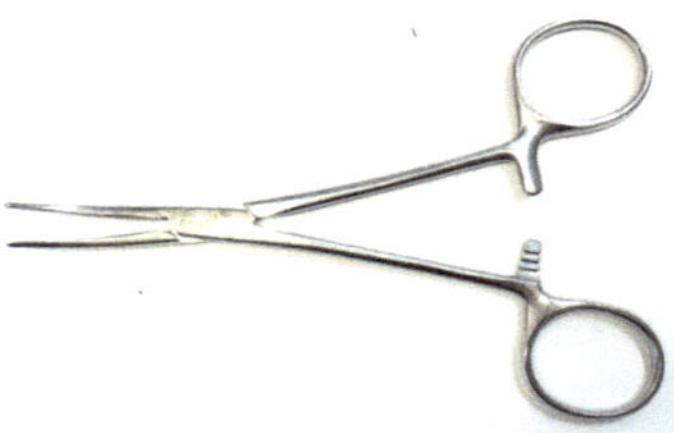

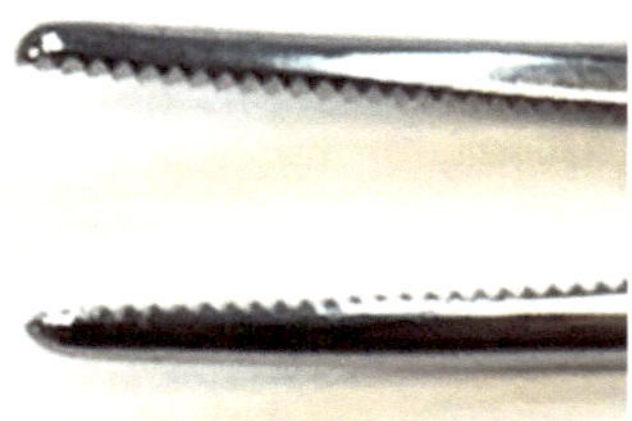

Roberts

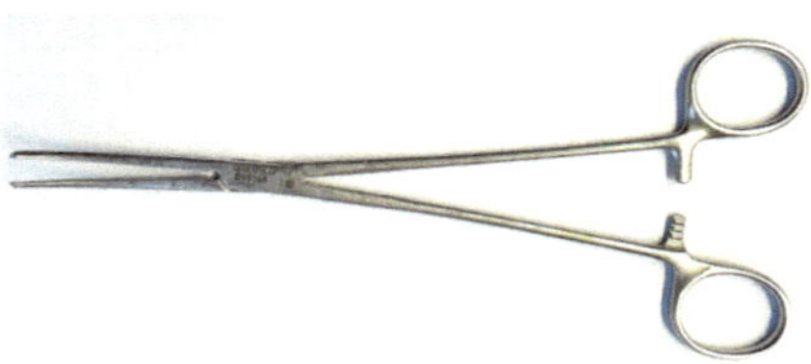

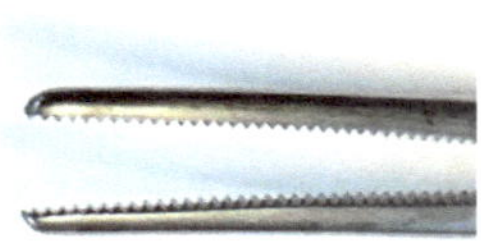

Moynihan

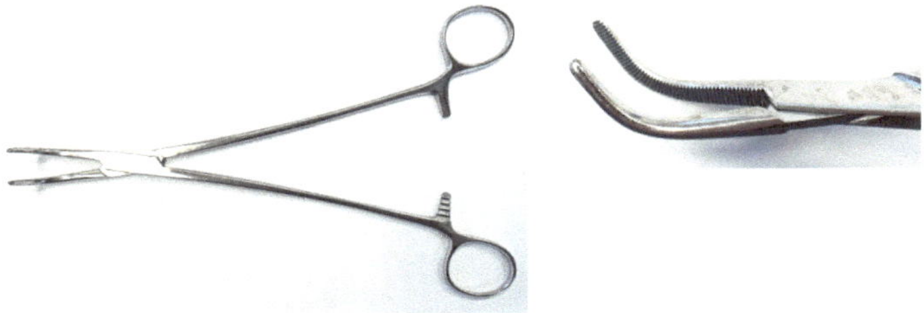

Green Armytage forceps

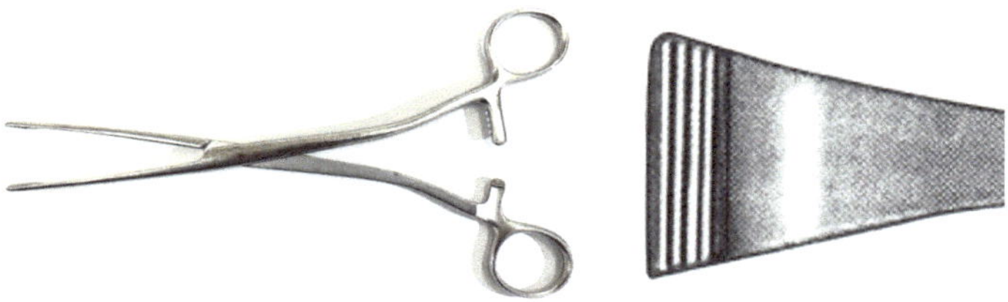

Right angle forceps

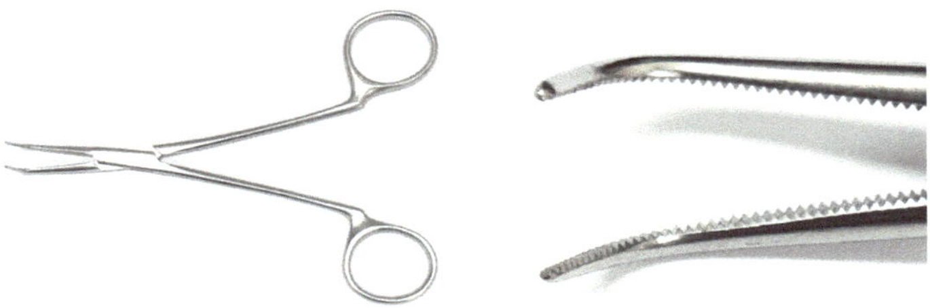

Hysterectomy clamps (Maingot, Heaney, Zeppelin etc)

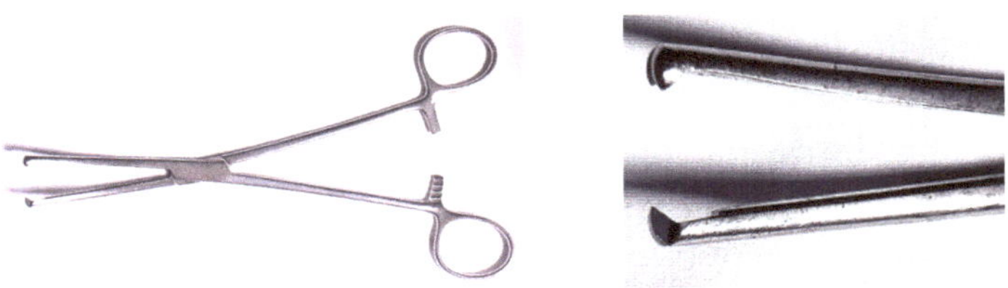

Haemostatic other

Vessel Clipper

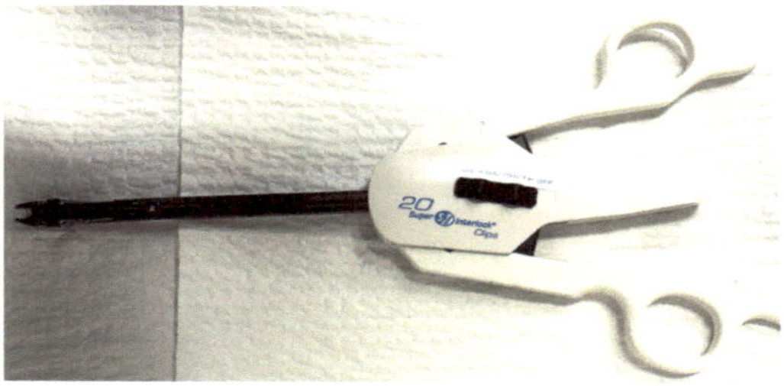

Retracting

Breisky retractor (also commonly called Braun retractor) (Various sizes)

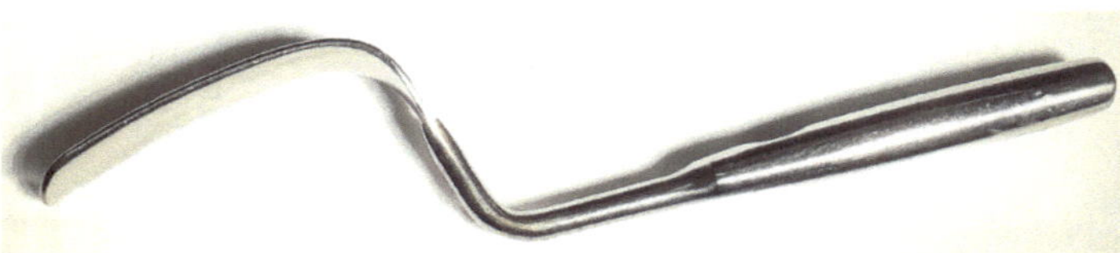

S retractor

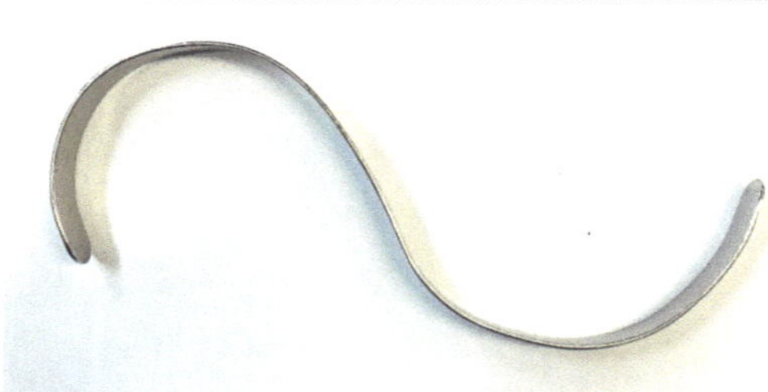

Langenbeck retractor (Various sizes)

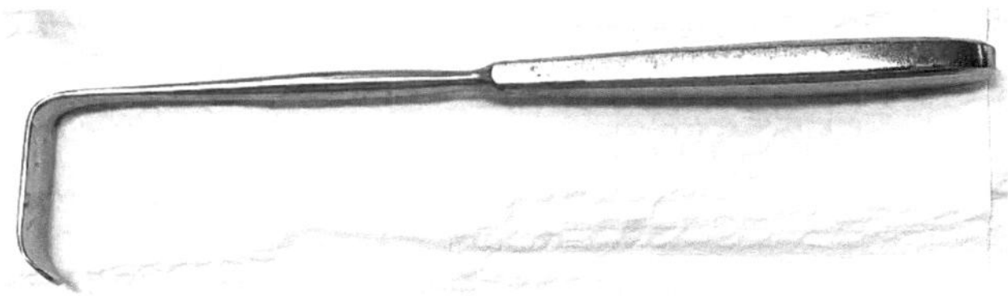

Army Paton (Army-Navy or American Paton) retractor (various sizes)

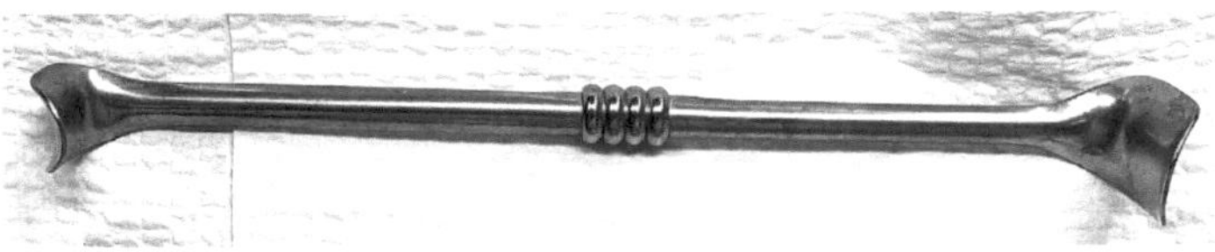

Canny Ryall & Durham retractors (essentially the same, but different handle grips)

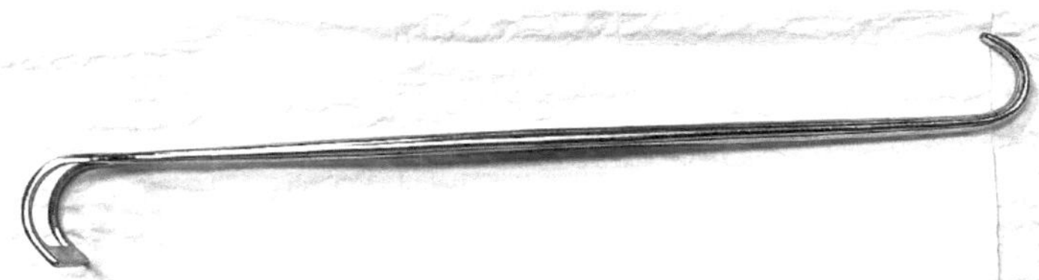

Deaver retractor (Various sizes)

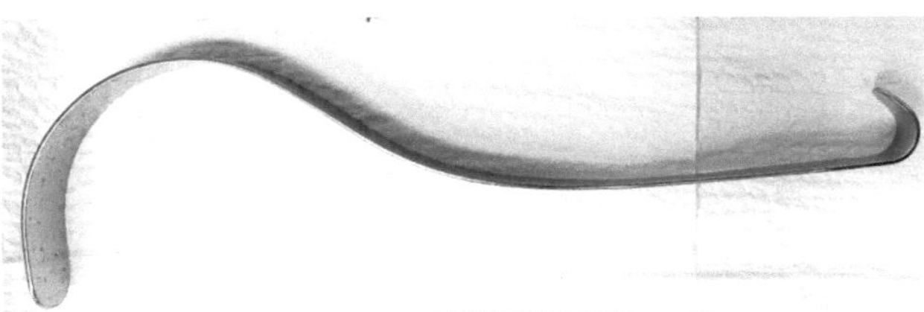

Right angled retractor (sometimes named Morrison's retractor)

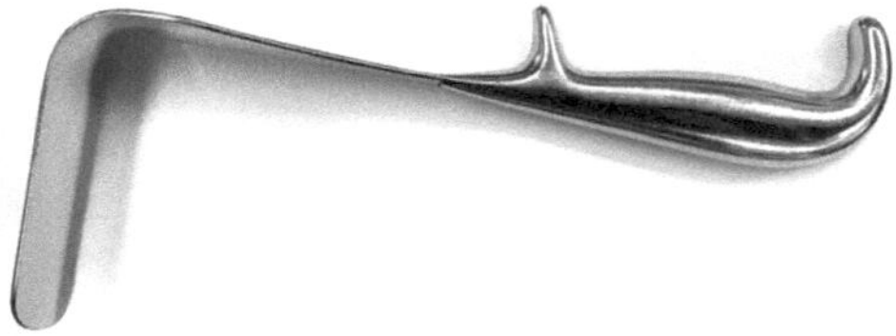

St Mark's retractor

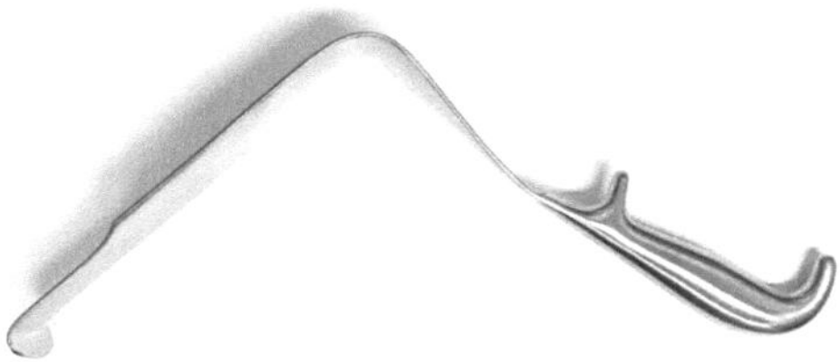

Fritsch bladder retractor

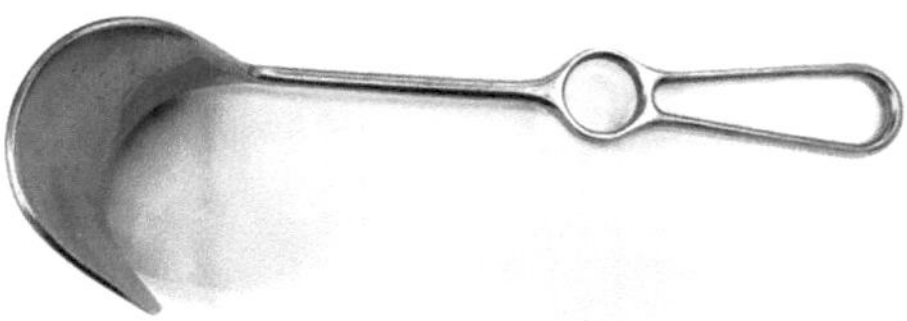

Cat's Paws

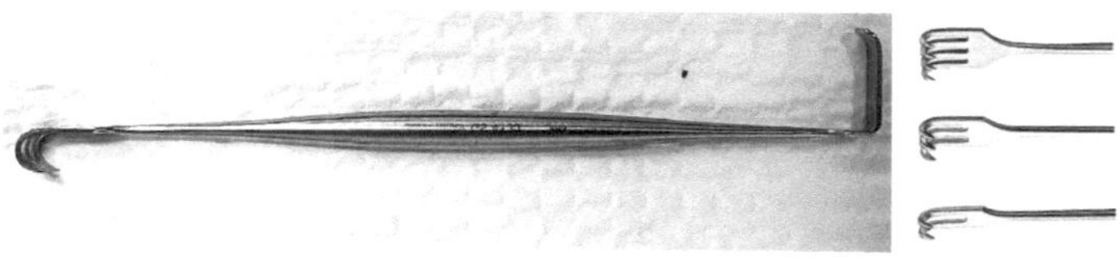

Skin Hooks

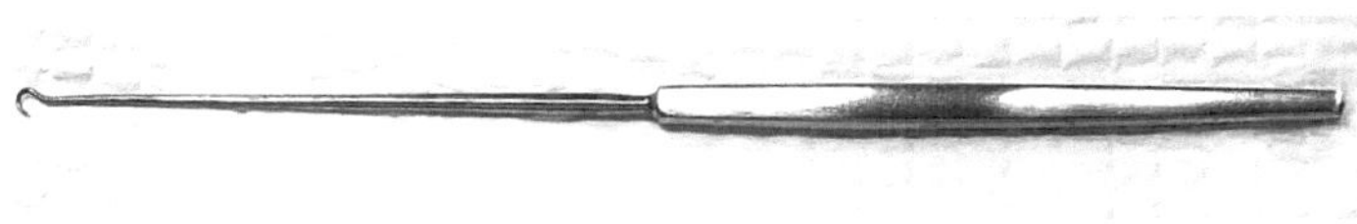

Self-retaining retractors

Mollison, Travers, Norfolk, Norwich, Weitlaner and Gelpie retractors (all similar but different sizes and number of retainers)

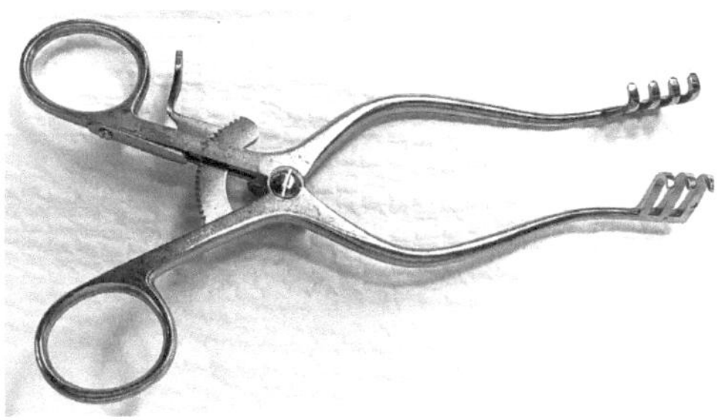

Balfour Doyen retractor

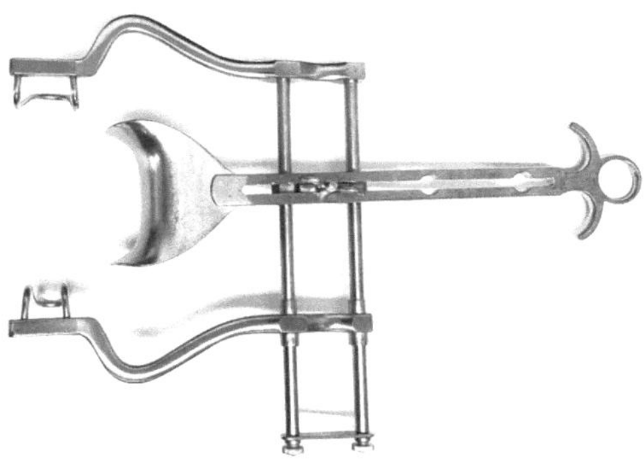

Bookwalter & various modifications including Thompson, Omni Tract retractors

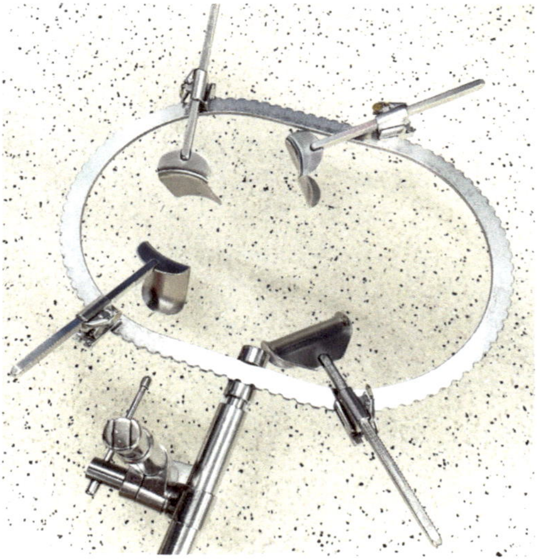

Lone Star retractor

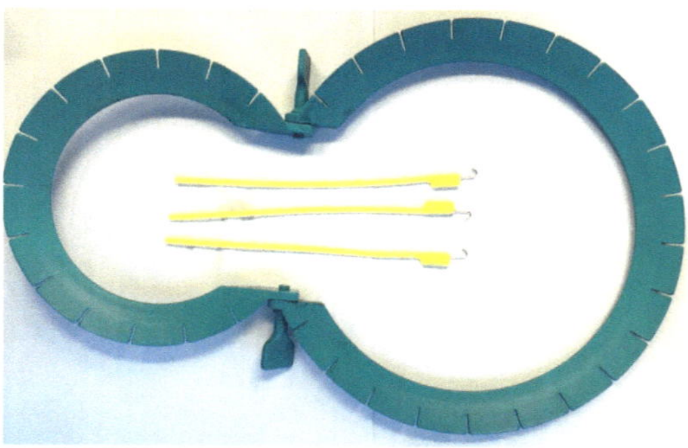

Alexis retractor - various sizes
(Caesarean Section type shown)

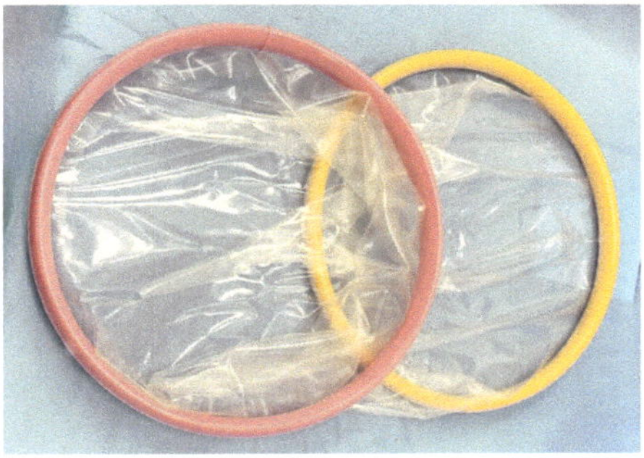

Cutting

Heavy: Mayo Scissors (curved or straight)

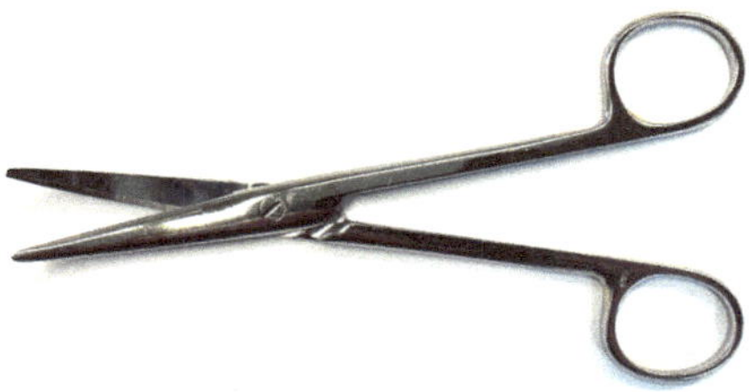

Light: Princess, Metzenbaum, McIndoe scissors
- all very similar (curved or Straight)

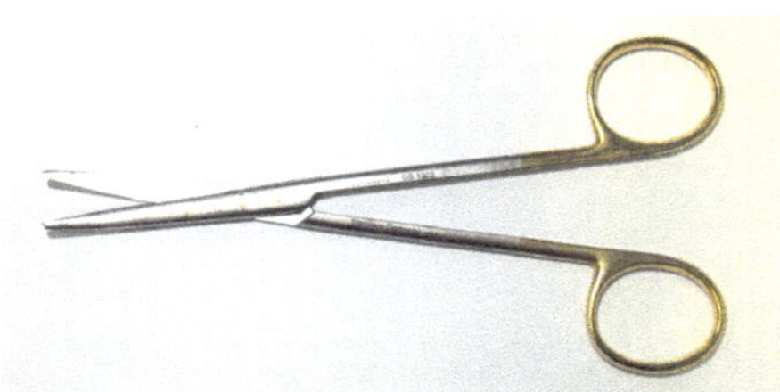

Tenotomy scissors

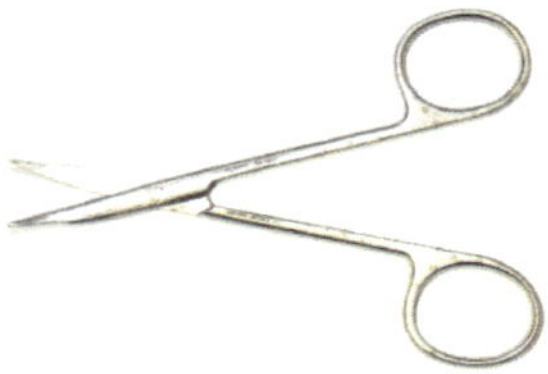

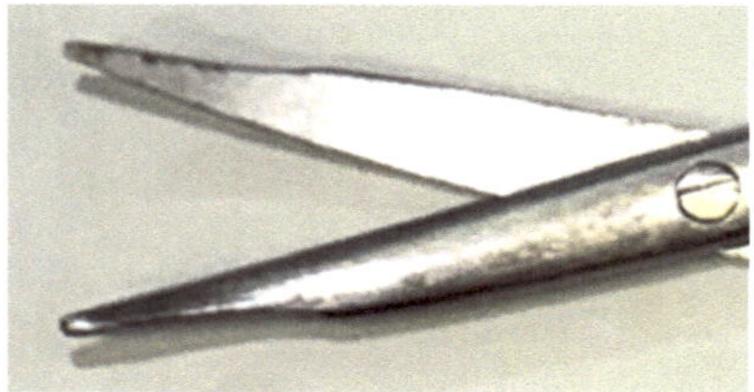

Suture cutting:

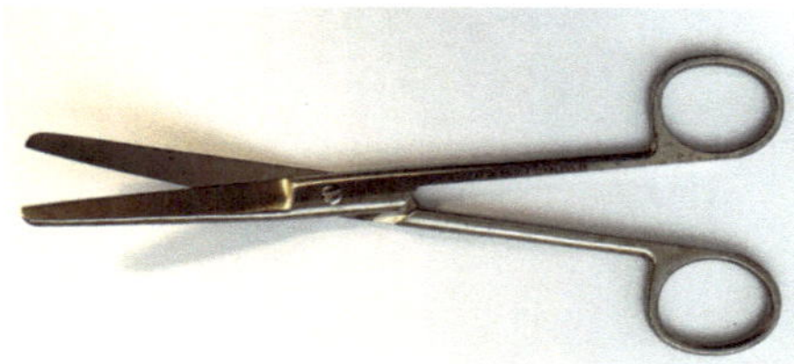

Suturing

Needle Holders

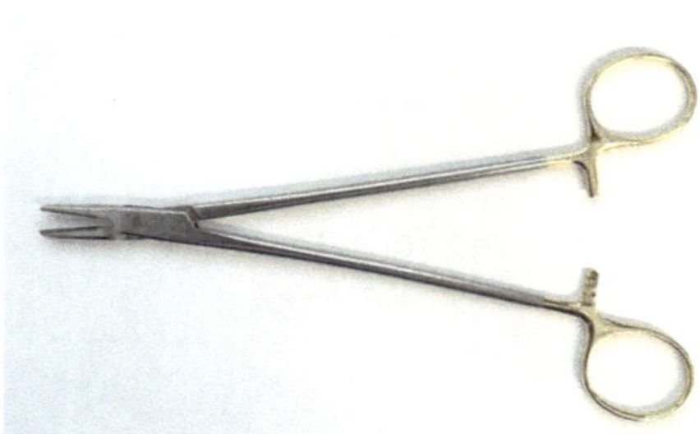

Suction

Yankauer sucker (metal or plastic)

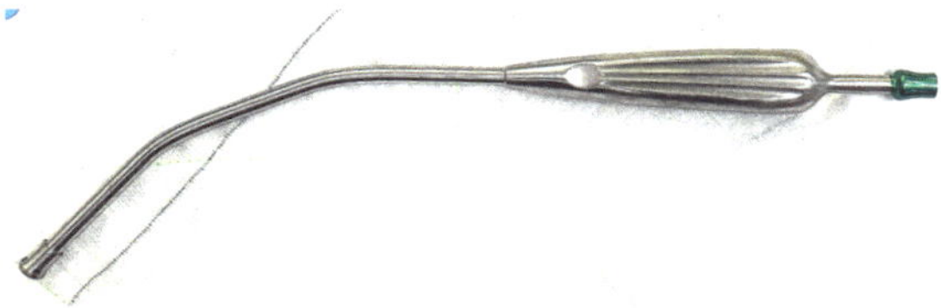

Simpson Sucker

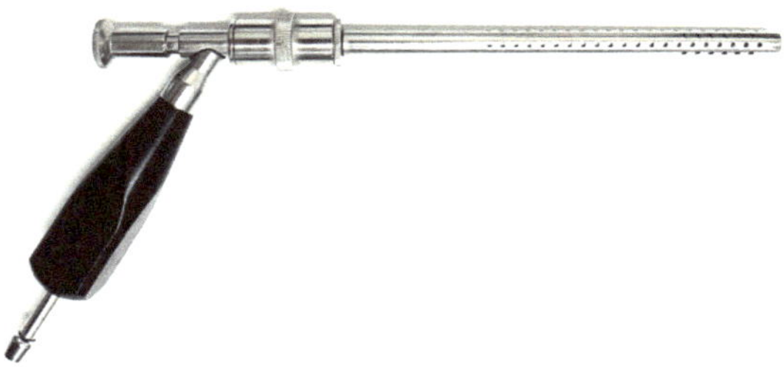

Energy devices

Handheld monopolar diathermy (shown with smoke evacuation)

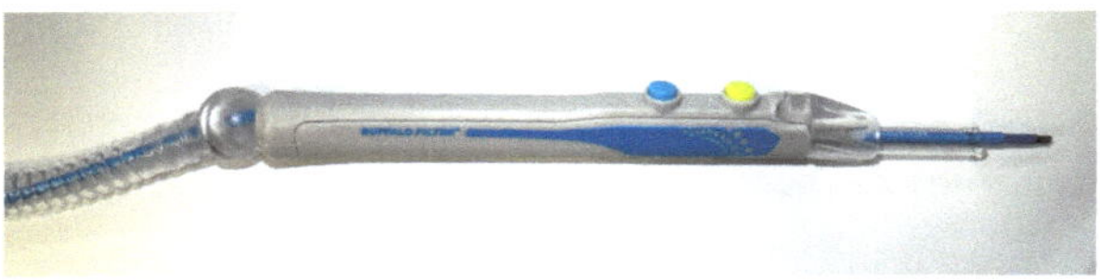

Handheld bipolar diathermy

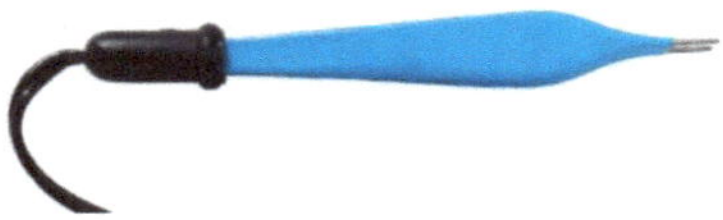

Skin staplers

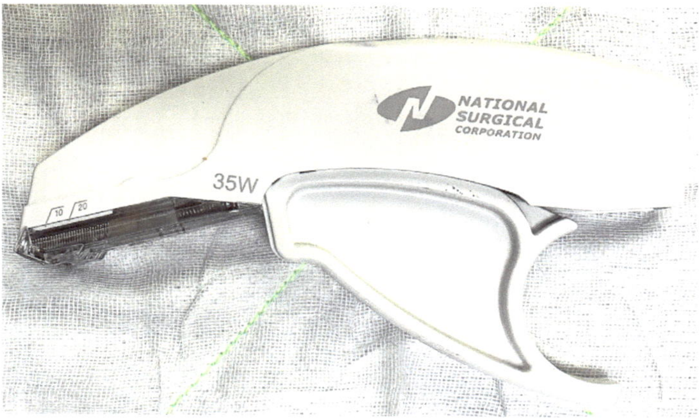

Endoscopic

Cameras and Scopes

Laparoscope, cystoscope, hysteroscope, arthroscope etc. with varying sizes and degrees of scope angle

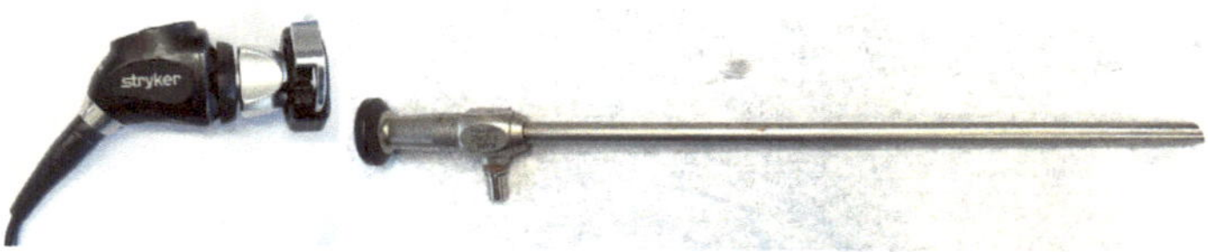

General Handles

Grasper handles (ratcheted)	Grasper handles (non-ratcheted)
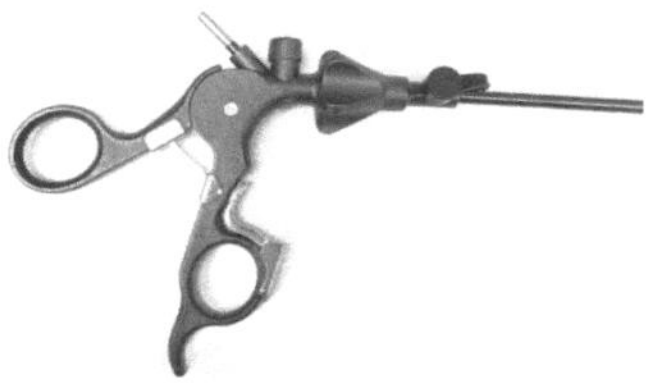	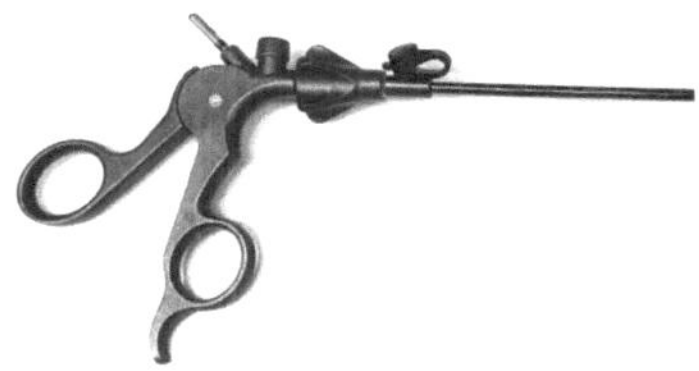

Tips

Maryland's forceps

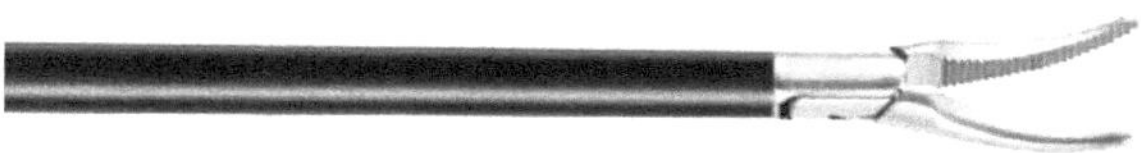

Toothed forceps

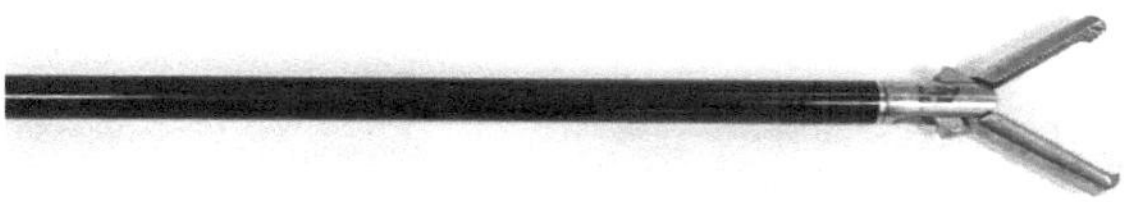

Fenestrated Forceps (Johan & others))

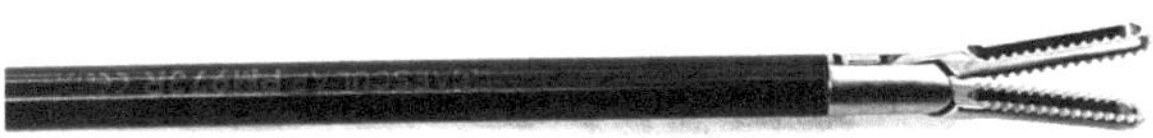

Atraumatic: De Bakey

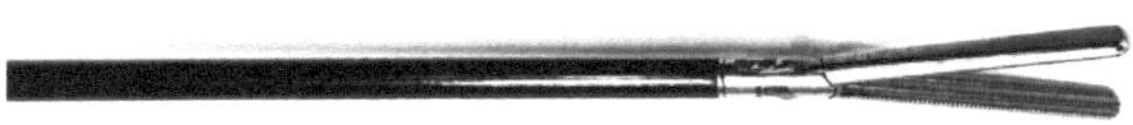

Atrac forceps

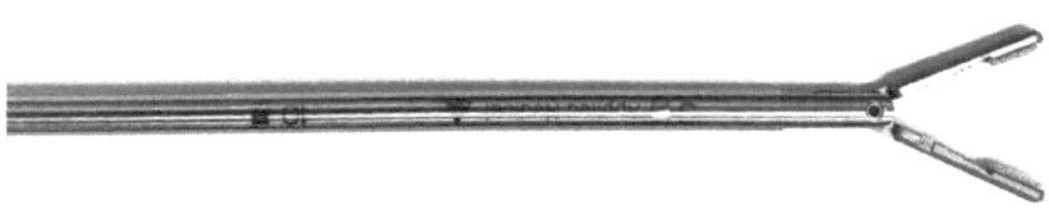

Needle holder

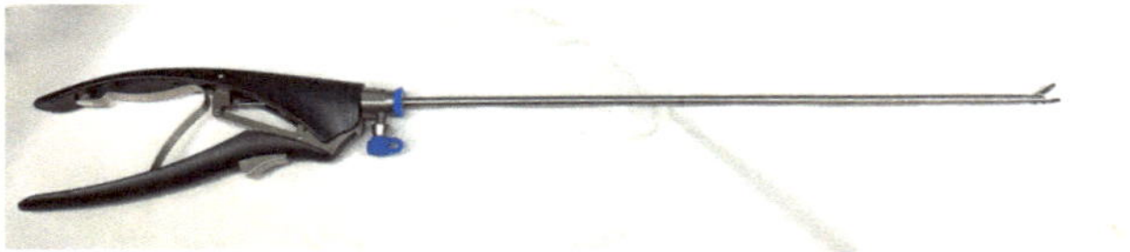

Scissors

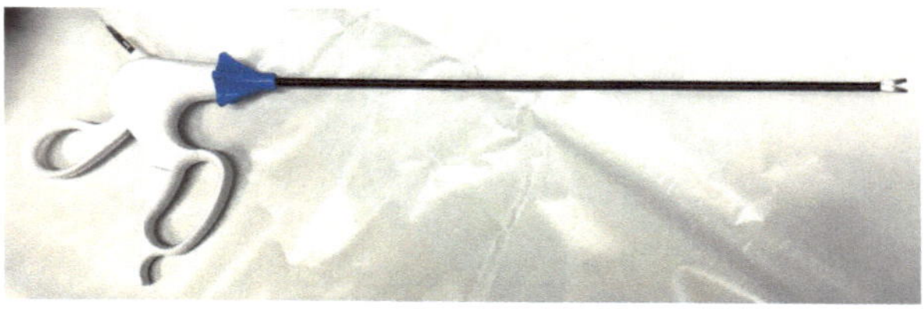

Energy devices

Monopolar spades and hooks

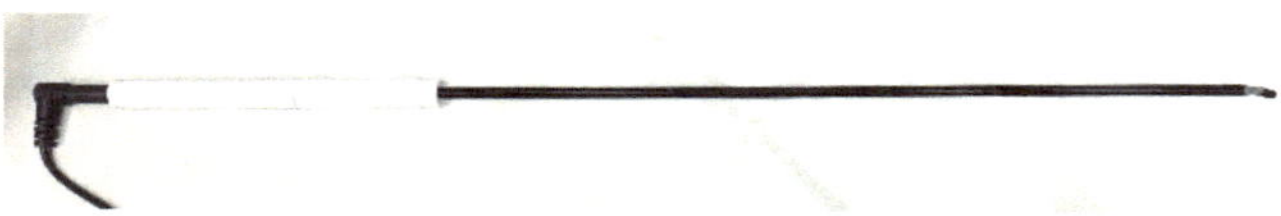

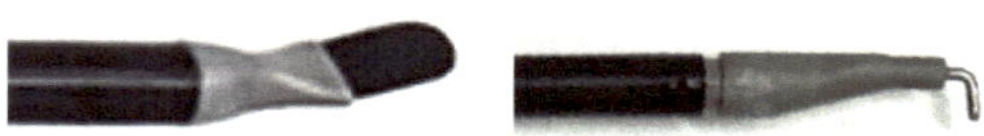

Bipolar diathermy devices (various e.g. Gyrus TM)

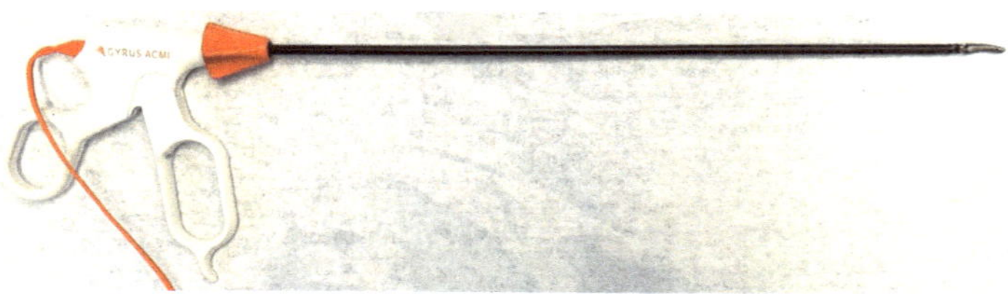

Combined bipolar and cutting (e.g. Ligasure TM)

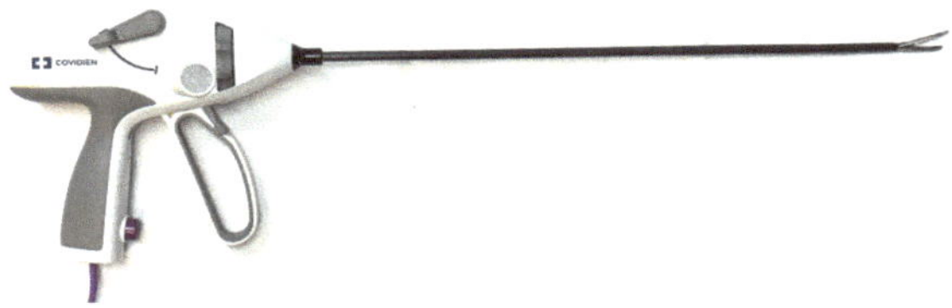

Combined bipolar & harmonic devices. Short versions for non-laparoscopic procedures (e.g. Thunderbeat TM)

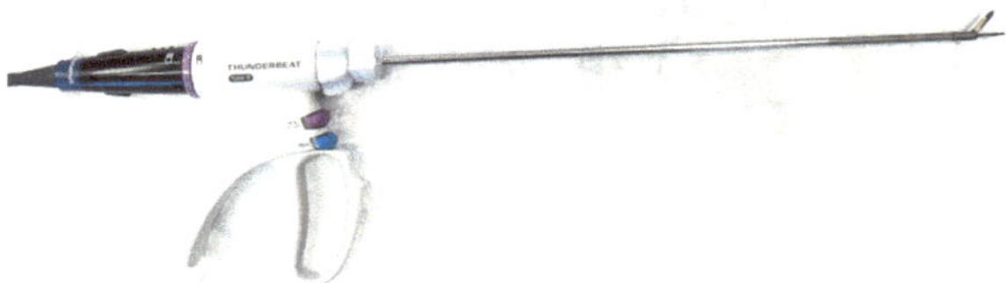

Haemostatic non energy

Endo Loop

Laparoscopic clipper

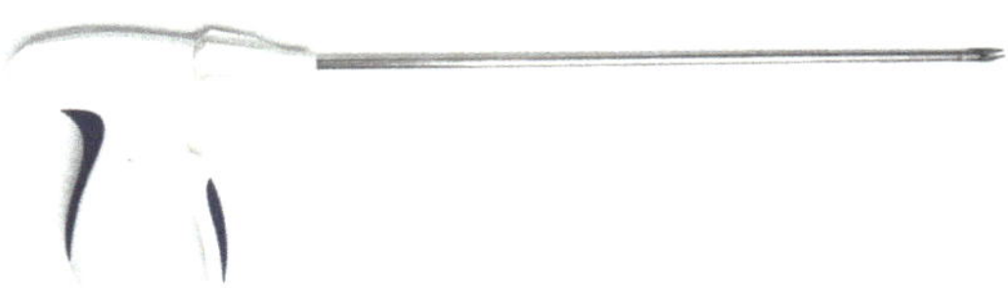

Suction devices

Laparoscopic sucker

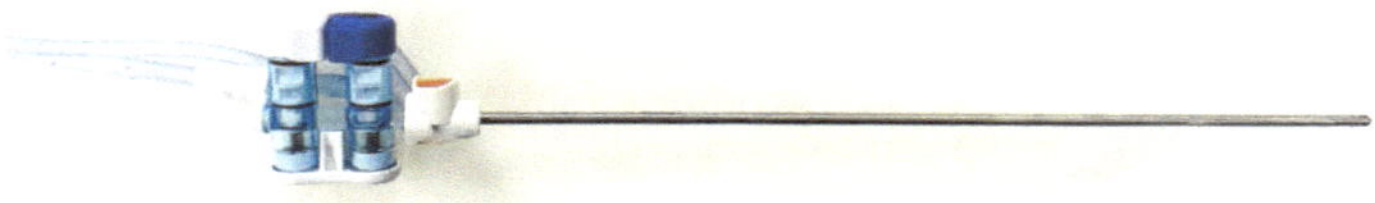

Retrieving devices

Endocatch^{TM} bag

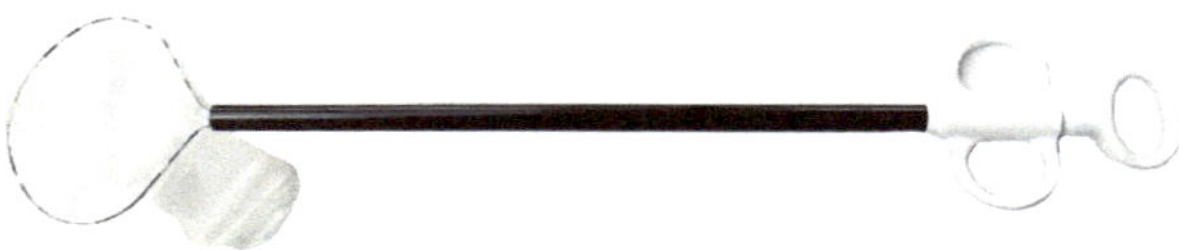

Specialised instruments

There are of course many more, such as various mallets, saws, drills, chisels, jigs etc in orthopaedics, staplers, sounds, probes, dilators, curettes, speculae, stents and catheters, drains and tubes etc. etc. in urology, gynaecology, colorectal, ophthalmological and neuro-surgery. These will become familiar with use if assisting in these areas.

BASIC SUTURE CHOICES & SUTURING TECHNIQUES:

The choice of suture and needle depends upon many factors such as tissue type, access, infection risk and often personal preference. As a surgical assistant you will usually be guided by the specialist surgeon. The following is simply a brief guide to provide some understanding as to why certain choices are made.

SUTURE CHOICES:

Sutures can be broadly classified using several criteria:

- Absorbable (broken down over varying time by enzymatic reactions or hydrolysis)
  Commonly used for rapidly healing and deep tissues such as small bowl anastomoses, repair of biliary and urinary tract and tying of small vessels near the skin. Absorption times vary for e.g. Vicryl Rapide TM ~42 days, Vicryl TM~60 days, Monocryl TM ~100 days, PDS~200 days

- Non absorbable. Commonly used for tissues that heal slowly and that require long term support. The sutures are usually walled off by the inflammatory process and may or may not need removal at some stage. e.g. for tendon or fascia repair, abdominal wall repair or vascular anastomoses.

- Natural: (e.g. silk or catgut) used less nowadays as they invoke a significant tissue reaction. Silk is sometimes still used for securing such things as drain tubes.

- Synthetic: (e.g. nylon or PDS) more predictable in their loss of tensile strength or absorption.

- Monofilament: (e.g. nylon, PDS or Prolene) lower infection risk but less ease of handling and less knot security.

- Multifilament (e.g. braided silk or Vicryl) ease of handling & good knot security, but increased infection risk.

Suture Type	Absorbable	Non-absorbable	Mono filament	Multi filament
Vicryl	*			*
PDS	*		*	
Monocryl	*		*	
Nylon		*	*	
Prolene		*	*	
Silk		*		*

Suture Size: the higher the number, the finer the suture (5.0 is thinner than 2.0). Tend to use the smallest size possible considering the nature of the tissue and the tensile strength required.

Needle size, shape and cut: these also vary depending upon the tissue being repaired, eg ***Round bodied*** for friable tissue such as liver and kidney, ***Cutting*** for penetrating tough tissues such as skin and bone, ***Reverse Cutting*** for tough tissues such as tendon or subcuticular tissue, ***Blunt tip*** for friable tissue and abdominal wall closure. Have less risk of needle stick injury. ***Sharp tip*** used especially where leakage is to be avoided.

The needle shape also varies in the proportion of a circle it forms (from 1/4 through to 5/8), depending on the ease of access to the area being sutured.
There are of course many more suture types including

knotless tissue control devices with a pre-formed "eye" and barbs for one-way continuous suturing (V-LockTM or StratafixTM brands for e.g.), wire "sutures" used in orthopaedics and many others.

BASIC SUTURING TECHNIQUES:

There are numerous online instruction videos that may also assist in learning suturing. **The aim is to approximate, not strangulate.**

The following are the most frequently used for skin closure:

- ***Simple interrupted:***

  The wound edge is generally stabilised with fine toothed (e.g. Gillies) forceps. To get good eversion and a better cosmetic result it is best to ensure the needle enters the skin in a perpendicular fashion about 4mm from the wound edge. This ensures a wider bite of deeper tissue than at the surface. The needle is continued across the wound and exits the skin in a similar fashion to the entry. (Figs. 1 & 2) The suture is competed by either an instrument or hand knot (see below).

Fig. 1

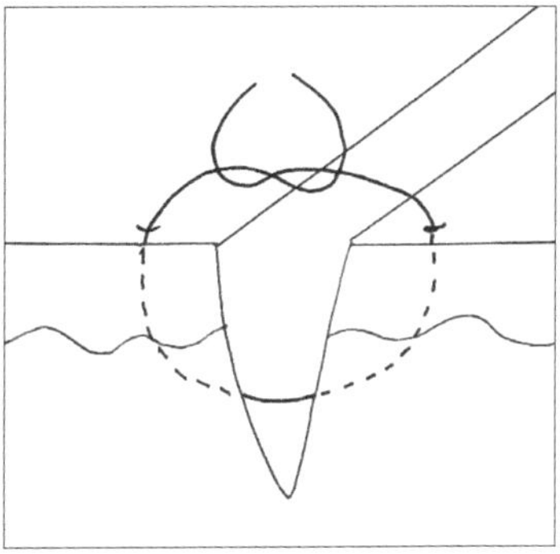

Fig. 2

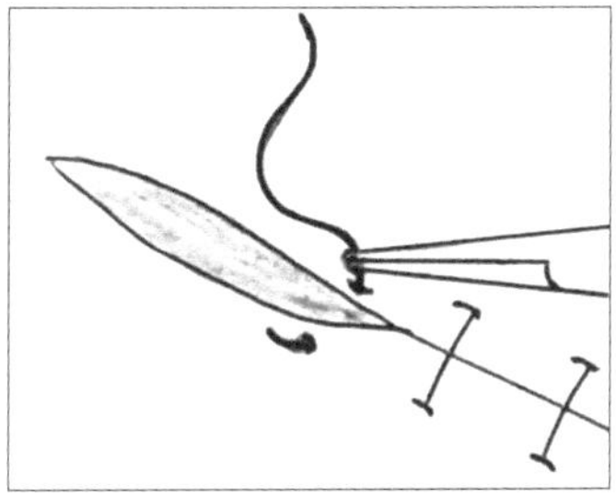

- ***Simple continuous running:***

  Whist this is time saving, scarring and ischaemia can be a problem, and the finished suture may not be as strong - if one part of the suture breaks, then the whole wound opens. If using this technique, an initial simple interrupted suture is performed at one end of the wound as above and leaving the needle end long to continue along the length of the wound. Once the end of the wound is reached a further knot is tied (e.g. instrument or hand knot).

Fig. 1

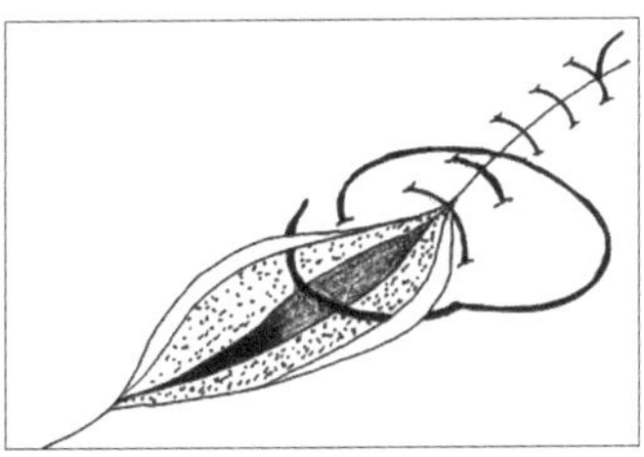

Fig. 2

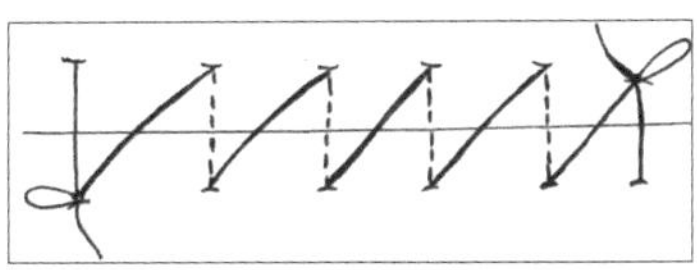

- ***Vertical mattress:***

  This suturing technique provides excellent support, wound eversion and less dead space. The needle is inserted 5-10mm. from the wound edge, a deep bite is taken, and the needle exits the other side of the wound at the same distance. The needle is then reversed in the holder and re-enters the 2nd side at about 3mm, a smaller bite is taken, and the needle exits the 1st side at about 3mm. (Figs. 1 & 2) A knot is tied to secure the suture._

Fig. 1

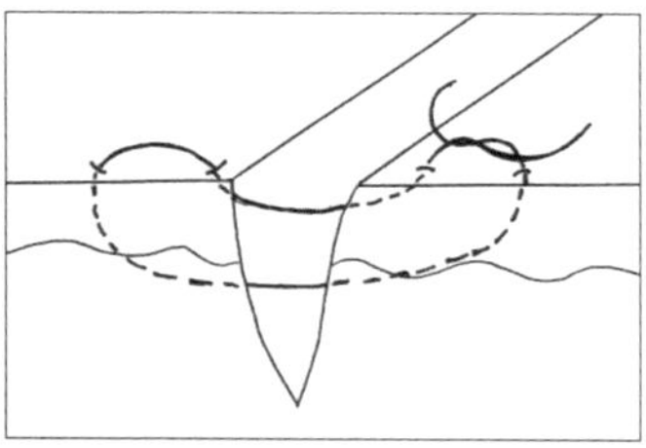

Fig. 2

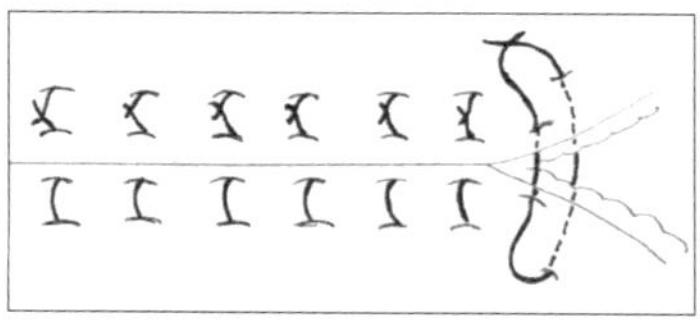

- ***Horizontal mattress:***

  If the wound is larger and there is a need to distribute the tension, then this suturing technique can be employed, even if only for the initial sutures. There is generally less ischaemia of the wound edges. The needle is inserted 5-10mm. from the wound edge, a deep bite is taken and then exits the 2nd side at the same distance. The needle then re-enters the 2nd side at about 3mm further along the wound, a deep bite is taken and then exits the first side also about 3mm along the wound. (Figs. 1 & 2) A knot is again tied to secure the suture.

Fig. 1

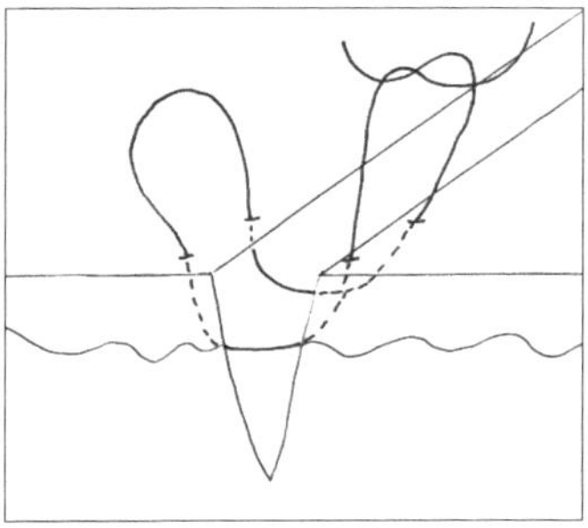

Fig. 2

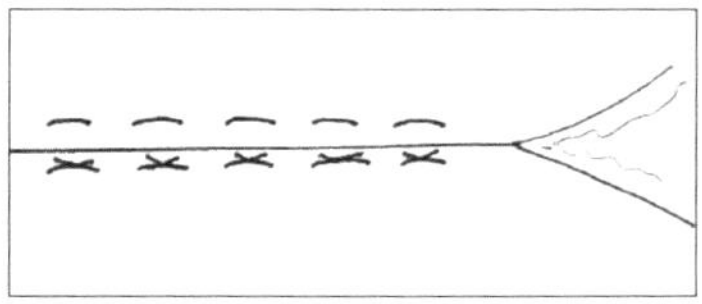

- ***Running locking (sometimes called a blanket stitch):***

  Useful especially if suturing under tension. The first suture is performed as per the simple interrupted above. The long (needle) end then completes the next suture, excepting that, before pulling taut onto the skin, the needle is inserted through the loop and locked. The process is continued along the length of the wound and a knot is again tied to secure the suture. (Figs. 1 & 2)

Fig. 1

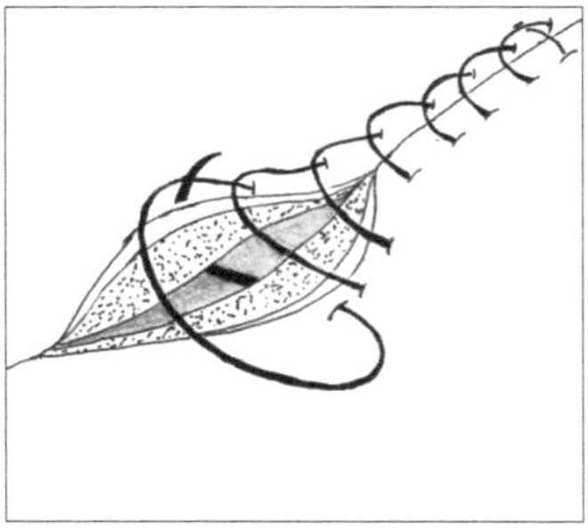

Fig. 2

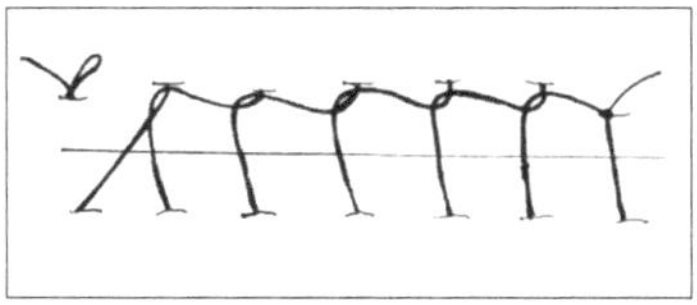

- ***Single Sub-cuticular:***

  This is useful for small incisions such as for small laparoscopic port entry incisions. It will be buried, so an absorbable suture such as fine monocryl is appropriate. The wound edge is everted with fine toothed forceps, the needle is introduced at the subcutaneous level and exits the same side at the dermal level. The needle then enters the dermal level of the 2nd side and exits at the same dermal level on this side. (Fig. 1). A knot is tied deep at the subcutaneous level and the free ends cut short to be buried. If a slightly longer closure is required (say 2 such sutures), the ends can be left long without tying an initial knot. A further pass is made as above, ensuring that the long (non-needle end) lies deep to the stitch. (Fig. 2). When completed, the knot can be tied, the needle passed out through the skin at the end of the wound, pulled tight, burying the knot and then cutting the non-needle end followed by the needle end at the skin surface.

Fig. 1

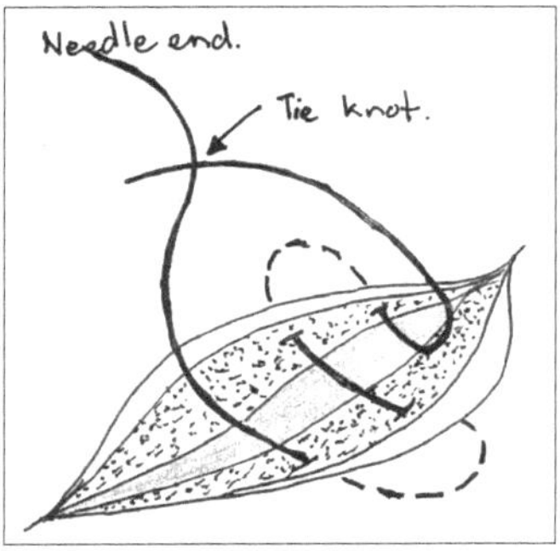

Fig. 2

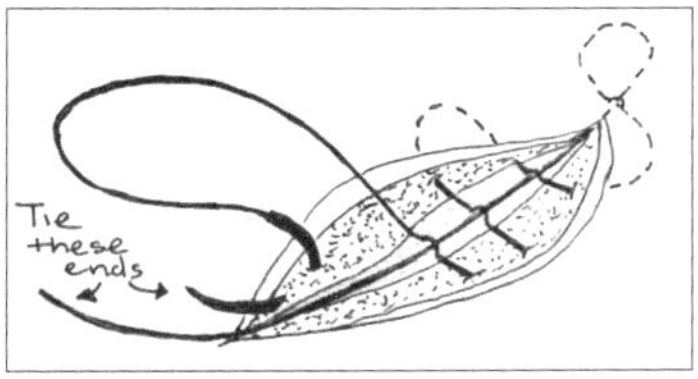

- ***Running Sub-cuticular:***
  This technique provides for less epidermal puncture points and therefore less scarring. The needle is introduced towards one end of the wound and a single sub-cuticular stitch is made and tied (as above). The long (needle end) is brought out the apex of the wound within the dermis (not through the epidermis). The short end is cut, and horizontal bites of dermis are taken from opposite sides of the wound in a "castle battlement" pattern (i.e. entering the dermis on one side immediately opposite the exit site on the other Fig. 2). This is continued along the wound to the other end, where a knot is tied

(Aberdeen knot, instrument tie or hand tie - the latter 2 will have one end as a loop which can be incorporated in the tie, but the Aberdeen is probably more suited). The needle then exits the epidermis just distal to this apex. (Figs. 1 & 2). The suture is pulled taut, burying the knot and cut flush with the skin.

Fig. 1

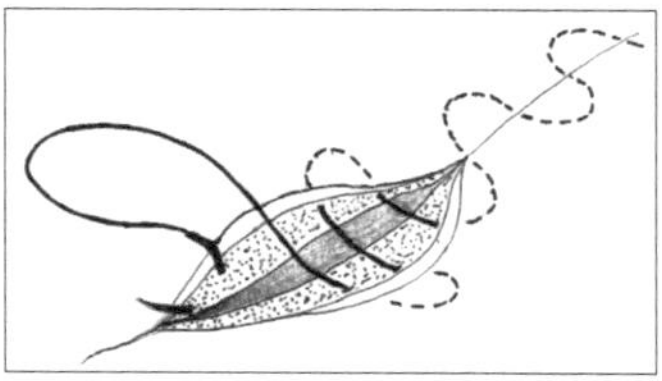

Fig. 2

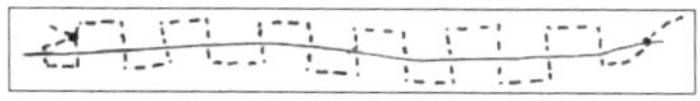

- SteristripsTM can be applied over the skin closures if appropriate

- Different special suturing techniques may be used for deep tissue closure (and are not discussed here).

- Some surgeons chose to use glues (HistoacrylTM, DemabondTM etc.) for smaller incisions.

- Some surgeons use staples for some skin closures.

BASIC KNOT TYING TECHNIQUES

In all suturing, some form of knot is required to secure the suture.

As with suturing, there are numerous online videos that may assist in learning knot tying. There are various knots that the surgical assistant may employ. These include for example:

- ***Simple instrument tie (square knot or surgeon's knot):***
  This is the most basic tie and can be used with any of the above suture techniques.
  Once the suture has been placed, keep a long (needle containing) and short end on each side of the wound. Twist the long end twice around the needle holder and grasp the short end with the needle holder (Figs. 1 - 2) and pull taut onto the opposite side of the wound to square the knot (Fig. 3). Whilst keeping the knot taut against the skin, repeat the turn around the needle holder, but for one turn only and in the opposite direction (Figs. 4 - 6). Repeat this up to about 4 throws alternating the direction each time. Cut the suture to length.
  This knot is also employed for intra-corporeal knot tying at laparoscopic surgery.

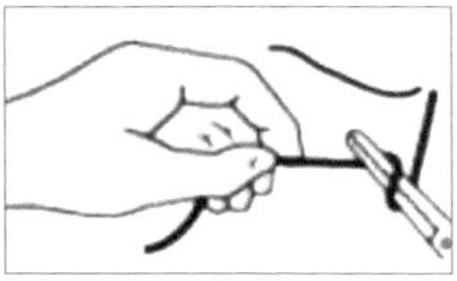
Fig. 1

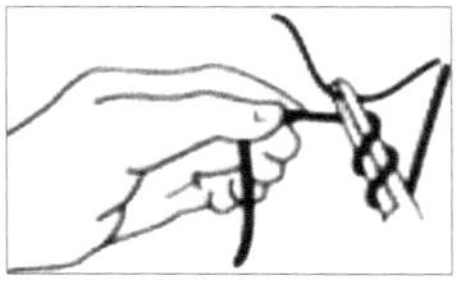
Fig. 2

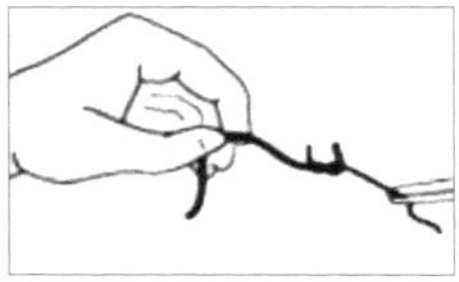
Fig. 3

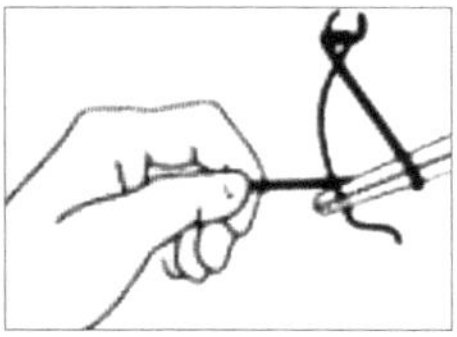
Fig. 4

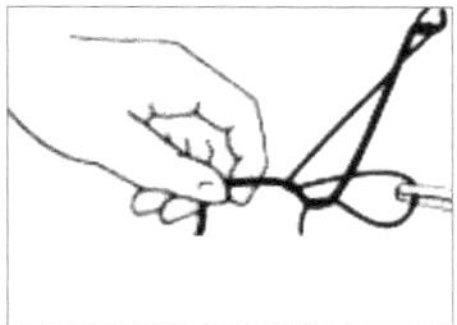
Fig. 5

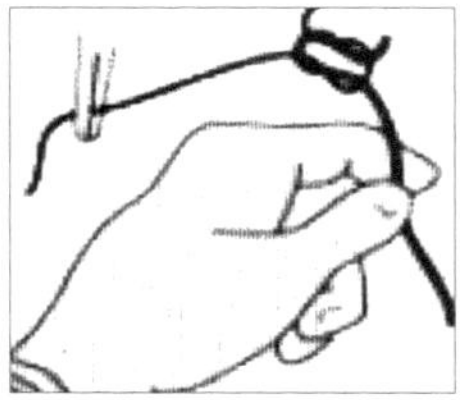
Fig. 6

- ***One hand surgical tie:***

  This is most useful when needing to suture deeper into a wound such as into the abdomen, where it is awkward to get the needle holder down deep into the wound. It can also be used in place of the simple needle tie for superficial wounds if preferred. There are numerous techniques described, and this is the technique that I have used throughout my career. The right hand which holds the needle and needle holder keeps this long end taut whilst the left hand does pretty much all the manoeuvring via the short end. This can of course be reversed if necessary for left hand dominant individuals.

  Once the suture has been placed, hold the long (needle containing) end taut in the right hand.

First throw: Grasp the short end between the thumb and index finger of the left hand (Fig. 1), and cross the short end over the long end, poking the left index finger through the loop made (Figs. 2 & 3) and hook the short end back through the loop with the left index finger (Fig. 4). Pull tight (Fig. 5).

Second throw: To reverse the direction of the above, grasp the short end between the left thumb and index finger, wrap it up over the middle, and ring and little fingers (Fig. 6). Now cross this over the needle end (which is in the right hand) over this to make a loop (Fig.7). Then grasp the short end between the left middle and ring fingers (steadying the loop with the left thumb) (Fig. 8), pull the short end through the loop (Fig. 9) and tighten (Fig. 10).

Repeat First and Second throws: as above and the knot is completed.
The ends can then be cut to length, or if using for skin closure of a buried suture, the needle end can be buried through the end of the wound, pulled taut and both ends cut at the skin surface (short or non-needle end cut first).

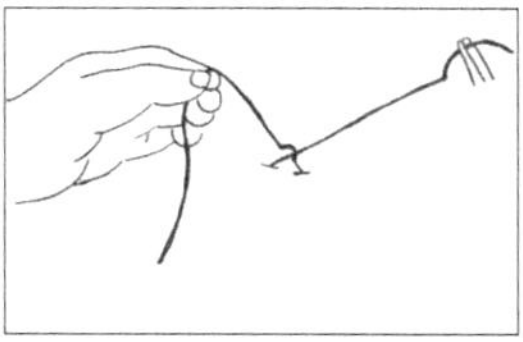

Fig. 1

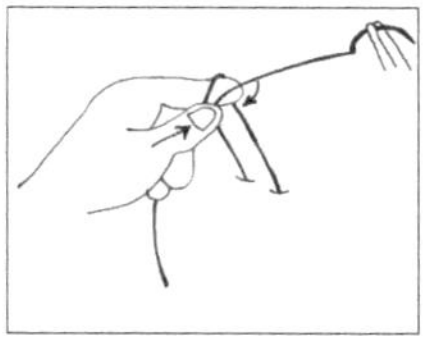

Fig. 2

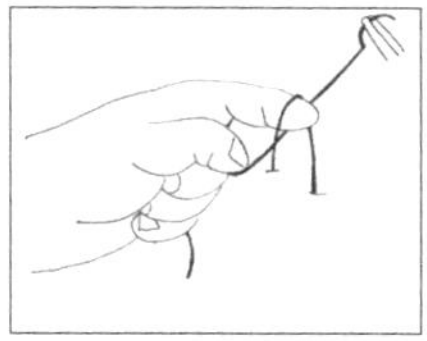

Fig. 3

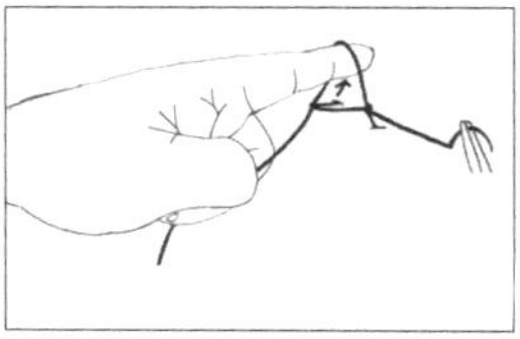

Fig. 4

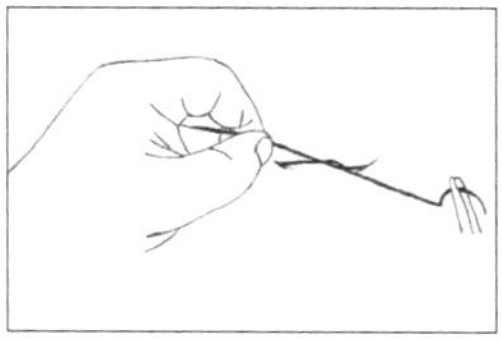

Fig. 5

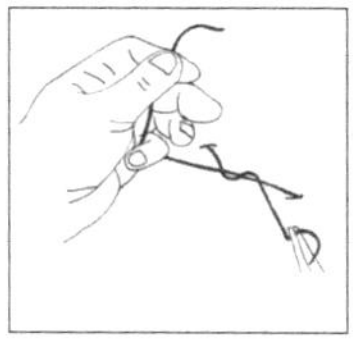

Fig. 6

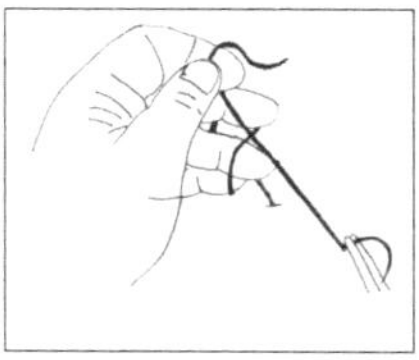

Fig. 7

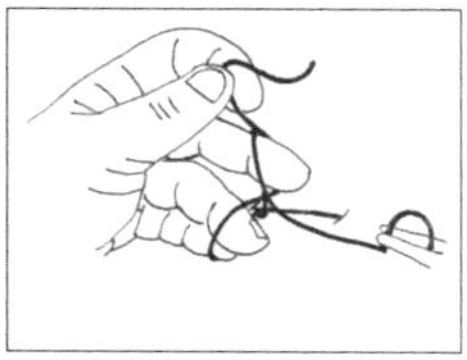

Fig. 8

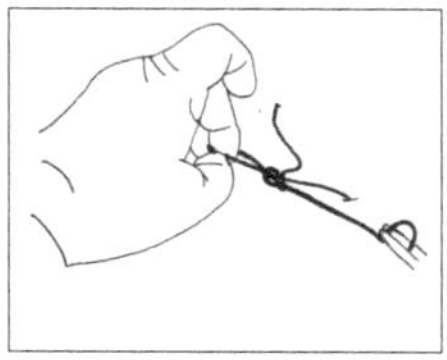

Fig. 9

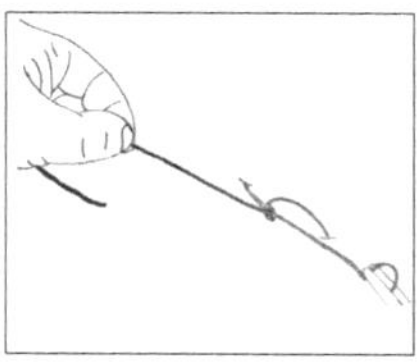

Fig. 10

- ***Various Specialised knots, such as:***

  Aberdeen knot:

  This is most useful for tying at the end of running sutures. It is stronger, more secure, less bulky than traditional square knots and, if needed, is easily buried.

At the end of the run keep out a loop and a long end (the needle end). Pass the fingers of the left hand through the loop keeping it close to the skin surface, grasp the long end with the left hand through the loop and tighten the loop down onto the long end whilst maintaining traction on this with both hands and forming another loop (Figs. 1-3). Repeat the above process for 4 throws using the newly formed loop each time. After these 4 throws, pass the entire long end including the needle through the final loop and pull taut to lock (Fig. 4). The suture can then be buried by inserting the needle through the apex of the wound and cutting at skin level.

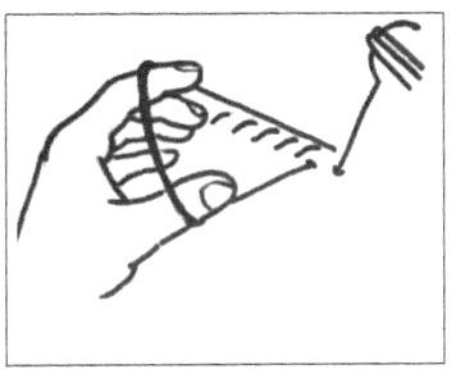

Fig. 1

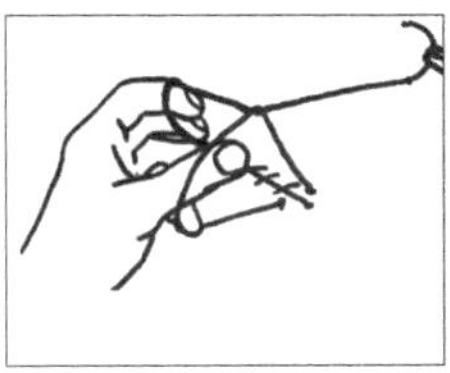

Fig. 2

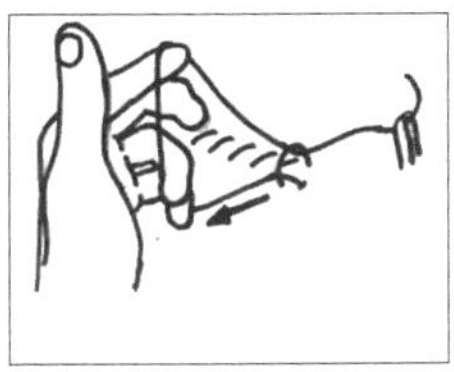

Fig. 3

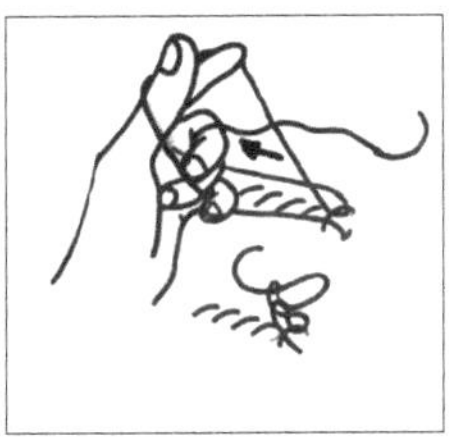

Fig. 4

- ***Modified Western knot:***

  This is a special knot that is particularly useful during laparoscopic surgery. It is tied extra-corporeally and due to its ability to slide, it is then slid down to the required site sometimes with a laparoscopic knot pusher or simply by pulling it taut. This is quite time saving as the simple square knot tie can be awkward at times using laparoscopic instruments.

  The needle end of the suture is inserted under vision down the port with an appropriate grasper. The non needle end remains out through the port. Once the suture has been placed around the intra-corporal structure, the needle end is drawn out through the same port and the needle cut off. Using 2 hands (and maybe an artery forceps) the knot is commenced:

  1. Equal lengths are grasped in each hand. The left-hand grasps one end between the flexed ring, middle and little fingers and the palm and looped over the extended and adducted thumb. The right-hand grasps the other end between the thumb and index finger (Fig. 1).

  2. The right-hand end is then draped over the left-hand end and left thumb (Fig. 2).

3. This initial right-hand end is then passed around through the loop formed (Fig. 3).

4. And around and back through this loop. (Fig. 4).

5. Rotate hand 90 degrees inwards (Fig. 5)

6. Now grasp the left pointing end between thumb and index finger and pull it through the loop now formed over the thumb. (Fig. 6)

7. Now pull this left end tight to form a knot. Hold right end (runner end) taut to allow knot to run down. Once knot is placed over site, (may use knot pusher to run down) cross ends over and apply extra tension to secure.

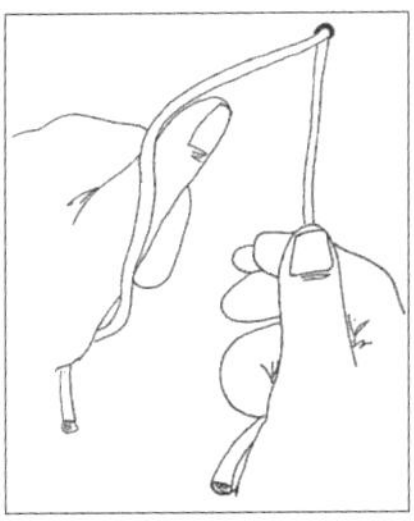

Fig. 1

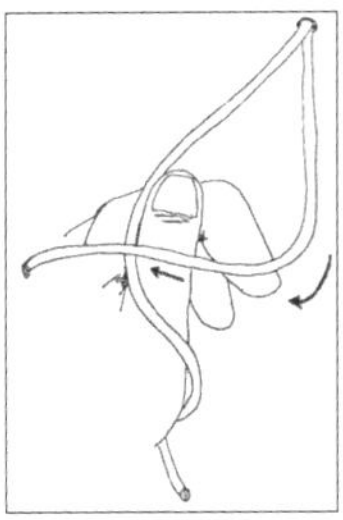

Fig. 2

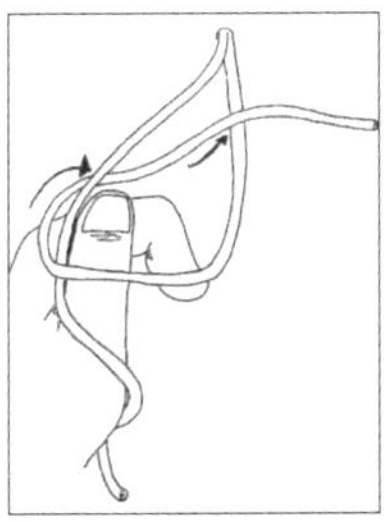

Fig. 3

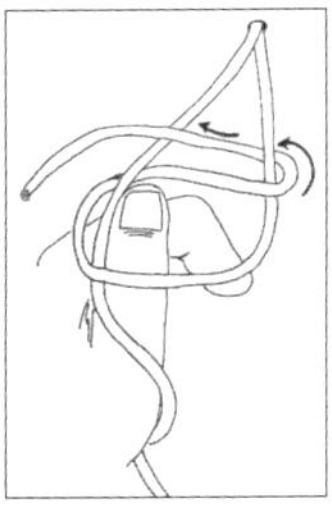

Fig. 4

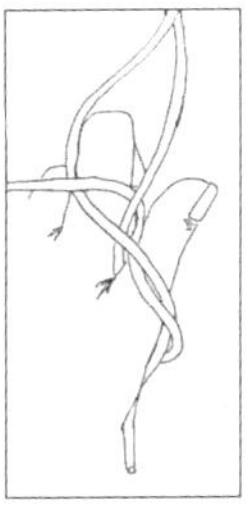

Fig. 5

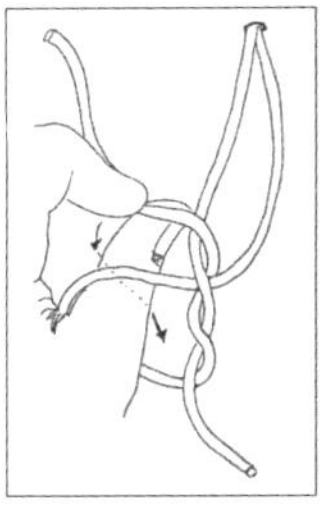

Fig. 6

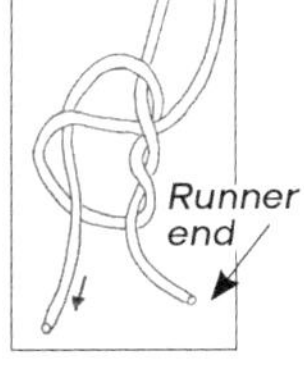

Fig. 7

BASIC URINARY BLADDER CATHETERISING TECHNIQUE

This is a common procedure that the surgical assistant may be expected to perform.

It is relatively simple to perform, but sterility and care are important. Generally, the patient will be anaesthetised or be under spinal anaesthesia when this is performed in the operating theatre.

Difficult catheterisations where for example rigid catheter introducers are required should not be undertaken by the occasional operator and should be performed only by those specifically trained and experienced in this technique.

Catheters come in a sterile pack, are usually gauged according to the external diameter of the tube and use the universal gauge as "French Size". The higher the number, the larger the catheter diameter. As a general guide: 6Fr, 8Fr and 10Fr are for paediatric, 12Fr and 14Fr are for adult female, 14Fr, 16Fr and 18Fr are for adult male and 20Fr and 22Fr are reserved for situations where clot retention is a potential issue.

- ***Female catheterisation:***
  Wash hands thoroughly and don sterile gloves. With the left hand part the labia & clean the area thoroughly using the right hand and a sterile swab holder with a sterile aqueous solution, paying particular to the urethral orifice. Drape the area, apply sterile lubricant to the catheter tip and insert the catheter with the right hand (avoid touching the catheter with the left hand as this has possibly been contaminated at the outset). Advance the catheter until urine flow is visualised and then advance a further 2 - 3 cm to ensure the balloon has passed the urethra. Inflate the balloon (usually 10ml), gently pull on the catheter to ensure that the balloon is in the bladder, and if not already connected, connect the sterile catheter bag. Ensure that the catheter is not putting tension on the urethra by securing it appropriately to the patient's thigh. Remove all drapes, syringes and swabs etc. Usually, a count of swabs will be undertaken. To remove the catheter, merely deflate the balloon with a 10ml syringe and extract the catheter.

- ***Male catheterisation:***
  Wash hands thoroughly and don sterile gloves. Clean the penis with a sterile aqueous solution.

Grasp the penis with the left hand, retract the foreskin if present to display the glans and urethral orifice, and further clean with the aqueous solution. Drape the area, apply sterile lubricant to the catheter tip, grasp the penis with the left hand, and raise it and insert the catheter with the right hand - advancing it from its sleeve (avoid touching the catheter with the left hand as this has possibly been contaminated at the outset). Once urine is obtained, advance a further 2-3 cm to ensure that the balloon has passed the urethra.

Inflate the balloon (usually 10ml), gently pull on the catheter to ensure that the balloon is in the bladder and if not already connected, connect the sterile catheter bag. Replace the foreskin if it has been retracted at the outset. Ensure that the catheter is not putting tension on the urethra by securing it appropriately to the patient's thigh. Remove all drapes and swabs etc. Usually, a count of swabs will be undertaken. To remove the catheter, merely deflate the balloon with a 10ml syringe and extract the catheter.

Note that in the male in particular, resistance can be encountered due to prostatomegaly. If this occurs and it cannot be overcome with gentle pressure and manoeuvring of the penis,

it is best to seek further advice from someone more experienced in this procedure.

Note also that if urine is not obtained (and if you're unsure if the catheter is in fact in the bladder or if the patient is dehydrated due to fasting), by attaching a sterile syringe to the sterile bag end of the catheter and applying gentle aspiration then some urine may be obtained to help solve this dilemma.

BASIC SCRUB TECHNIQUE

There are numerous online modules that describe this, and many hospitals have posters in the scrub area outlining the procedure, but nothing really surpasses being shown in person. The following is a general outline of the procedure. ***Remember if you're not sure then swallow your pride and ask someone to show you the correct procedure.***

- Ensure that you are wearing the correct attire - Surgical scrubs (bare below the elbows without watches or jewellery), theatre head wear, comfortable, closed washable footwear (clogs) or disposable over boots.

- Fit a surgical mask with appropriate eye protection. Ensure this is comfortably fitted as you cannot adjust this once scrubbed.

- Proceed to the scrub sink, open packaging containing the small scrub sponge with nail brush and nail pick, place these on the edge of the sink still in the package, start the running water (either by electronic eye, foot or elbow controls), wet the hands and arms and apply the sterile scrubbing solution (betadine TM, or chlorhexidine) working up a lather from fingers to elbows.

- Rinse thoroughly, keeping elbows bent and hands above allowing water to flow from fingers to elbows.
- Using nail brush and nail pick clean under nails as indicated. Dispose of these without touching anything else. Keep elbows bent to allow water to flow from fingers to elbows
- Apply water and sterile scrubbing solution to palms and thoroughly work this in between all fingers of both hands. Allow the water and solution to run down to elbows.
- Scrub one arm at a time (down to elbows) and always keep hands above elbows.
- Rinse and repeat, this time down to mid forearms.
- Rinse and repeat, this time for fingers, hands and wrists - again always keeping hands above elbows.
- With hands still above elbows (and away from face), proceed to operating theatre, opening the doors using your feet, backside or electronic no touch openers pending the hospital.

- Proceed to gowning up table (which the scrub nurse has usually set up with appropriately sized gloves, gown and sterile towel. Keep hands above elbows still.

- Pick up corner of sterile towel with one hand and use one side to dry the opposite hand.

- Then place this side of the towel into the dried hand and use the other side of the towel to dry the opposite hand. Keep hands above elbows still, and you're ready to gown and glove. (see below)

Note if at any time, the procedure breaks down (such as touching anything other than the above) then the whole process will need to start again.

Note also that many hospitals now also allow the use of a dispensable alcohol solution or gel (e.g. Skinman TM) which allows a somewhat shorter scrub technique, but the basic principles of obtaining and maintaining sterility still apply. This is now becoming the usual technique according to ACORN standards. (see poster on facing page, provided with permission from Ecolabs, re use of this technique)

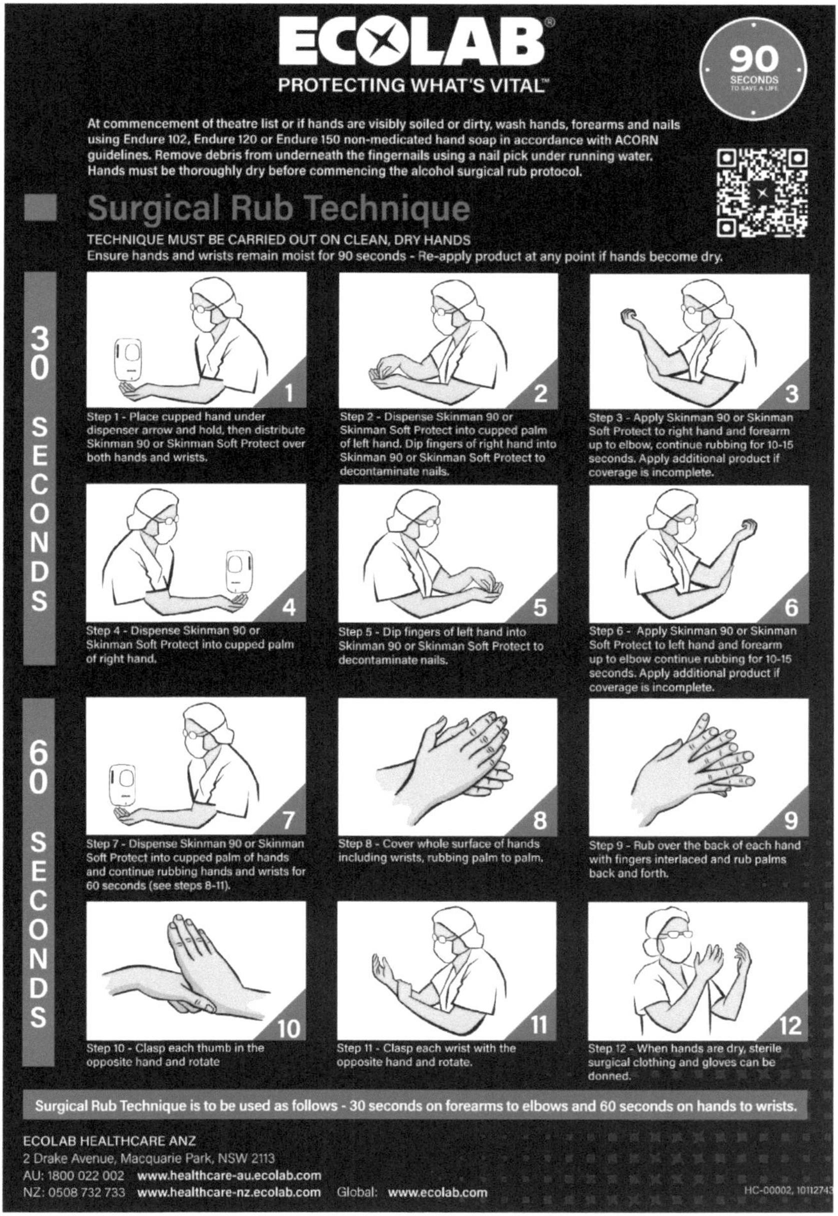
ECOLAB®
PROTECTING WHAT'S VITAL™
90 SECONDS TO SAVE A LIFE
At commencement of theatre list or if hands are visibly soiled or dirty, wash hands, forearms and nails using Endure 102, Endure 120 or Endure 150 non-medicated hand soap in accordance with ACORN guidelines. Remove debris from underneath the fingernails using a nail pick under running water. Hands must be thoroughly dry before commencing the alcohol surgical rub protocol.
Surgical Rub Technique
TECHNIQUE MUST BE CARRIED OUT ON CLEAN, DRY HANDS
Ensure hands and wrists remain moist for 90 seconds - Re-apply product at any point if hands become dry.
30 SECONDS
Step 1 - Place cupped hand under dispenser arrow and hold, then distribute Skinman 90 or Skinman Soft Protect over both hands and wrists.
Step 2 - Dispense Skinman 90 or Skinman Soft Protect into cupped palm of left hand. Dip fingers of right hand into Skinman 90 or Skinman Soft Protect to decontaminate nails.
Step 3 - Apply Skinman 90 or Skinman Soft Protect to right hand and forearm up to elbow, continue rubbing for 10-15 seconds. Apply additional product if coverage is incomplete.
Step 4 - Dispense Skinman 90 or Skinman Soft Protect into cupped palm of right hand.
Step 5 - Dip fingers of left hand into Skinman 90 or Skinman Soft Protect to decontaminate nails.
Step 6 - Apply Skinman 90 or Skinman Soft Protect to left hand and forearm up to elbow continue rubbing for 10-15 seconds. Apply additional product if coverage is incomplete.
60 SECONDS
Step 7 - Dispense Skinman 90 or Skinman Soft Protect into cupped palm of hands and continue rubbing hands and wrists for 60 seconds (see steps 8-11).
Step 8 - Cover whole surface of hands including wrists, rubbing palm to palm.
Step 9 - Rub over the back of each hand with fingers interlaced and rub palms back and forth.
Step 10 - Clasp each thumb in the opposite hand and rotate
Step 11 - Clasp each wrist with the opposite hand and rotate.
Step 12 - When hands are dry, sterile surgical clothing and gloves can be donned.
Surgical Rub Technique is to be used as follows - 30 seconds on forearms to elbows and 60 seconds on hands to wrists.
ECOLAB HEALTHCARE ANZ
2 Drake Avenue, Macquarie Park, NSW 2113
AU: 1800 022 002 www.healthcare-au.ecolab.com
NZ: 0508 732 733 www.healthcare-nz.ecolab.com Global: www.ecolab.com
HC-00002, 1011274

BASIC GOWNING & GLOVING TECHNIQUE:

Traditionally the scrub nurse "gowned and gloved" the surgeon, but this is now the exception, and we are generally expected to gown and glove ourselves. Again, there are numerous online resources describing this, but nothing surpasses first hand observation and instruction for this. This too is merely a general outline of the procedure.

Again, remember if you're not sure then swallow your pride and ask someone to show you the correct procedure.

- ***Gowning:***

    - Whilst maintaining sterility, with one hand pick up the folded gown from the "gowning & gloving" table and then with both hands ensure that you have a grip on all layers and that you are holding the gown from the inside only.

    - Step back from the table, hold the inside firmly and allow the gown to unfold downwards, whilst ensuring that neither you nor the gown touch any other unsterile objects.

- Grasp the insides of the shoulders, open the gown (inside facing you) and insert one arm into each arm hole at a time. Stop short of extending your hands through the cuff and grasp the inside seam of each cuff between the thumb and index finger of each hand.

- An un-scrubbed theatre staff member will then secure the back of your gown (unsterile area).

♦ ***Gloving:***

- With your hands still inside the arms and not protruding beyond the cuffs, pick up the right glove with your left hand and place it palm down on the right hand which is palm up.

- Place the glove so that the thumbs line up with yours, but the glove is facing toward you i.e. opposite to your hand. The folded edge of the glove should be at the level of the seam of the gown cuff.

- With the left hand which is still in the arm of the gown grasp the right glove and roll it over the right hand. Grasp the right glove cuff and sleeve with the left hand and pull these fully onto the right hand and pull any excess cuff out of the glove.

- Using the right hand that is now gloved, put on the left glove in the same manner as the right-hand glove.

- Ensure that there isn't any excess of cuff out of the glove and adjust the fingers of both so that they fit comfortably.

- Maintain sterility - keep hands between chest and waist and don't touch anything unsterile

♦ ***Turning (Final tie):***

- Locate the cardboard tab at the front of the gown at about waist level. It holds a long and a short tie together.

- Detach the short tie and hold it in your left hand. Hold the tab and the connected long tie in your right hand.

- Without touching the un-scrubbed staff member (or anything else unsterile), pass the tab and the long tie to them.

- With their guidance turn allowing them to pass the tab and long tie around your back

- Grasp the long tie (not the cardboard tab). The un-scrubbed staff member will tear the tab off without touching the long tie.

- You now have two ties which you can tie in a bow at the front at your waist.

- You are now completely gowned and gloved with appropriate sterility.

Remember to maintain sterility. Do not touch anything that is unsterile (including your mask or gown above your chest or below your waist). If you don't know what to do with your hands, then either keep your hands together in front of your chest or cross your arms across your chest. If you breach sterility, admit it and appropriate measures can be taken to correct this. It takes some time for all of this to become 2nd nature. Even after over 40 years of doing this, I still occasionally breach sterility by mistake at times and must correct it. So do almost all specialist surgeons.

BASIC REQUIREMENTS FOR SETTING UP PRIVATE BILLING (IN AUSTRALIA):

The following is a practical guide if you intend to do your own billing and applies to the situation in Australia (some Australian state requirements may vary in some details).

- **PRODA:** Register with PRODA (Provider Digital Access). This can be done through the Australian Government's Services Australia website.
- **Provider number:** This can be done online through PRODA.
- **ABN:** Check with your accountant as you may already have an ABN. This can otherwise be acquired through the Australian Government's Australian Business Register website
- **Accreditation:** Apply for accreditation at each individual surgical site
- **Email Address:** It is advisable to set up a designated email address for all correspondence relating to this surgical assistance.

- **Postal Address:** A Post Office Box (or surgery address if you have one) is advisable as a preferred method of receiving information or cheques (when necessary), particularly from patients.

- **Residential (or other) Address:** Some health providers will not accept a Post Office Box for sending statements, or cheques (when necessary). These are posted to nominated practice address (i.e. residential or other address listed for the provider number). You may request that a residential address not be given to patients or made public. (It is advisable not to have a hospital address as the main address, as correspondence is not always delivered, or can be misplaced - especially for cheques).

- **Bank Account:** A Credit Card Account is not accepted

- **Phone Number:** It may be preferable to have a separate mobile phone number for patients to contact you when necessary.

- **Registration with Private Health Funds:** All Private Health Funds can be found through Australian Government's Services Australia website.

- **Registration with the Motor / Road Accident / Workplace Injury Schemes:** All relevant departments can be found through each Australian State's Government website. These will differ between Australian States.

CLAIMING REQUIREMENTS for Medicare and Private Health Funds (in Australia):

- **Patient Details:** Full name, Date of Birth, Postal Address, Email Address, Phone Number(s).

- **Medicare Number:** Full Medicare Number including Reference Number and expiry date. (Parent's name, date of birth and Medicare number required if patient is under 18 years of age).

- **Private Health Fund:** Private Health Fund details and member reference number (Parent's name, date of birth and Medicare number required if patient is under 18 years of age).

- **Surgeon:** Full Name, address and Provider Number.
- **Site of Surgery:** Hospital / Day Surgery Site and Provider Number.
- **Date of Surgery:**
- **Item Number(s):** Surgeon will advise item number or combination of item numbers applicable to the procedure. NB: If assistance is required at a combination of two surgeons on a single patient, you will also need times specified and item numbers from both surgeons and specified on account(s).
- **Patient Out of Pocket (Gap):** Most health funds stipulate that any Out of Pocket / Known Gap charged to the patient, must be stated on the account.

CLAIMING Through Medicare and Private Health Funds (in Australia):

- **Medicare Benefits Schedule:** "MBS Online" is available through Australian Government Department of Health and Aged Care website.

- **Medicare:** Uninsured patient claims can be made through PRODA via bulk bill and patient claiming site.

- **Private Health Funds:** Most Private Health Funds have their own Batch Header to be used for claiming. These can be downloaded through individual health fund sites. (Many funds have their own list of fees, available for download).

CLAIMING REQUIREMENTS for Motor / Road Accident / Workplace Injury Scheme (in Australia & vary between States):

- **Patient:** Full Name, Date of Birth, Address, Phone Number.

- **Employer:** Name, Address, Phone Number, Contact Person.

- **Date of Injury:**

- **Injury Description:**

- **Claim Number:**

- **Insurance Company:** Claims Manager, Address, Contact Number.

NOTE: *As each country has their own hospital claiming practices, private health fund details can be found through the individual country's Government website.*

It is also worth noting that when a surgeon requests an assistant, a surgical assist item number will be associated with the surgeon's item number (denoted by "(Assist)" in the Medicare Schedule of Fees).

Unfortunately, not all surgical item numbers will have an assist item attached, but assistance is requested by the surgeon.

In this instance, discussion and clarification with the surgeon prior to the procedure is advisable. The suggestion is to discuss a fee that may be appropriate to either charge directly to the patient (advising the patient that a rebate is not available from Medicare), or alternatively for the surgeon to pay for the assistance. This can be facilitated by obtaining the theatre operating list with quoted item numbers in advance.

It is not appropriate for the assistant to be expected to perform their duties without remuneration.

ABOUT THE AUTHOR:

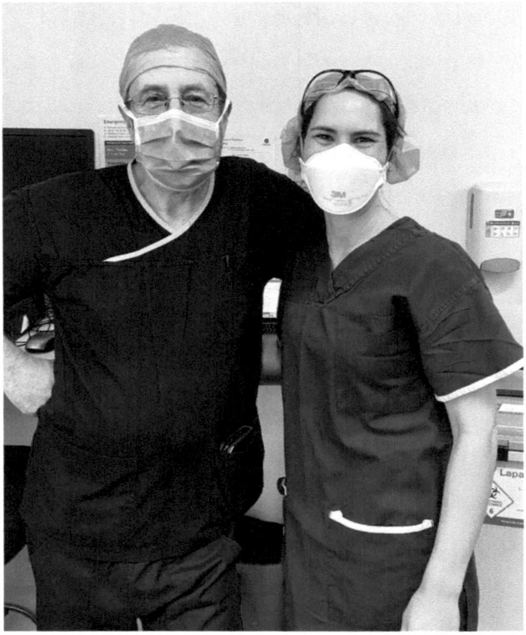

Dr Leeton Hocking & Dr Madeleine Ward

Leeton Hocking was born in Ballarat Australia in 1957. He was educated in Ballarat and graduated from the University of Melbourne with Bachelor of Medicine and Surgery in 1982. After graduation, he worked in the public hospital system for several years and obtained his Diploma of Obstetrics from the then Royal Australian College of Obstetricians and Gynaecologists in 1986.

He subsequently entered Family Medical Practice (General Practice) and continued as a General Practitioner / Obstetrician for many years. He maintained his passion for surgery by continuing to assist numerous specialist surgeons whilst also continuing to practice family medicine.

Over the years he has assisted many surgeons from various disciplines including Obstetrics and Gynaecology, General Surgery, Colorectal Surgery, Thoracic Surgery, Breast and Reconstructive Surgery and Orthopaedic Surgery. Throughout this time, he has assisted with the training of medical students, and registrars in both Family Medicine and the various surgical specialties.

Since 2024 he has retired from Family Medicine and continues to practice entirely as a surgical assistant at facilities in Ballarat and Geelong in Victoria Australia.

He is married and has two adult sons.

www.ingramcontent.com/pod-product-compliance
Lightning Source LLC
LaVergne TN
LVHW051129210926
848482LV00001B/33

* 9 7 8 1 7 6 4 4 2 8 2 1 7 *